CHANGING SEASONS
Macrobiotic Cookbook

OTHER AVERY BOOKS ABOUT MACROBIOTICS:

American Macrobiotic Cuisine
Meredith McCarty

The Macrobiotic Approach to Cancer
Michio Kushi with Wendy Esko

The Macrobiotic Cancer Prevention Cookbook
Aveline Kushi with Wendy Esko

The Macrobiotic Community Cookbook
Andrea Bliss Lerman

The Macrobiotic Way
Michio Kushi

Making the Transition to a Macrobiotic Diet
Carolyn Heidenry

CHANGING SEASONS
Macrobiotic Cookbook

Cooking in Harmony with Nature

Revised and Updated

Aveline Kushi and Wendy Esko

AVERY

a member of Penguin Group (USA) Inc.

New York

AVERY

a member of
Penguin Group (USA) Inc.
375 Hudson Street
New York, NY 10014
www.penguin.com

Library of Congress Cataloging-in-Publication Data

Kushi, Aveline.
The changing seasons macrobiotic cookbook : cooking in harmony with
nature / Aveline Kushi and Wendy Esko.—[Updated ed.].
p.   cm.
Includes index.
ISBN 1-58333-164-6
1. Macrobiotic diet—Recipes.   I. Esko, Wendy.   II. Title.

RM235.K85   2003   2003040383
641.5'63—dc21

Printed in the United States of America
11   13   15   17   19   20   18   16   14   12

Book design by Amanda Dewey

Acknowledgments

We would like to thank the people who inspired and contributed to this cookbook.

We would like to thank Michio Kushi for guiding so many people toward health and happiness as the basis for the future peaceful world, for inspiring the creation of this book, and for contributing an introduction.

We also thank Edward Esko for helping to edit and coordinate the text, and for conceiving the general orientation of the book. We extend appreciation to Alex Jack for editing the final draft, and thank Olivia Oredson and her associates for compiling notes and recipes from cooking seminars at the Kushi Institute.

We also thank Bill Tara, director of the Kushi Foundation in Brookline, for helping to arrange publication of the book; and Steve Blauer, Rudy Shur, Diana Puglisi, and Avery for their guidance and efforts.

Our deepest gratitude goes to George and Lima Ohsawa, who pioneered the macrobiotic approach and introduced it to millions of people throughout the world.

Finally, we thank all of you who read and use this cookbook in preparing daily meals. May it serve you in continuing health and happiness.

Aveline Kushi
Wendy Esko

Contents

Foreword

Winter is coming to an end and spring is just beginning as we complete this new cookbook. The snow has melted away and the spring rain becomes warmer with each day. We can see crocuses emerging from the ground and blooming. The grasses are becoming greener and the sweet smell of spring is in the air. This is a very wonderful and enjoyable sight to see.

This past winter, we decided to write a simple cookbook with recipes for each of the four seasons. We hope that this new book will be helpful in preparing meals for your family and friends. The recipes presented here are not fancy or special. In fact, they are generally those that we cook and serve in our homes from day to day. It is very nice to enjoy special holiday or party-style dishes occasionally, but for our daily food, we generally serve simpler and less fancy dishes.

The Kushi family consists of five children, two daughters-in-law, and four grandchildren. Wendy and her husband also have eight children. We daily serve the dishes presented in this book to our families, and we are living happily without any major problems or troubles.

The quality of the raw materials is very important when you cook for health and happiness. High-quality natural and organic foods are the ideal ingredients for daily use. They are the building blocks for a healthy and happy life.

For the single person, the macrobiotic way of eating may seem a little expensive. But if you carefully note the cost of items such as meat, processed foods, vitamins, and supplements—which are completely unnecessary when you eat whole natural foods—you will find that, in the long run, this way of eating is much less expensive. At the same time, the cost of medications, which is often quite high, can be substantially reduced or eliminated as a result of the improved health that comes from eating high-quality, properly prepared whole foods. The macrobiotic way of life is actually quite economical when all these considerations are taken into account.

Both of us have written other macrobiotic cookbooks and feel that this new book complements them very nicely. We have made this book very practical and easy to use. Included are many new recipes and some of the latest cooking techniques taught by Aveline and other instructors at the Kushi Institute. The approach presented in this book stems from common sense and the intuitive ability to harmonize our diet with the natural rhythms of change. Adapting to our changing environment is very important if we are to maintain a healthy and happy life. We hope that *The Changing Seasons Macrobiotic Cookbook* can help guide you in this endeavor.

At the Kushi Institute we teach a variety of cooking styles, including home-styled cooking, cooking for cancer and other illnesses, traditional food processing, institutional food preparation, and international cooking. Classes are given by a staff of teachers who have all had many years of experience in cooking under a wide variety of circumstances. Most of our teachers also cook for their families on a daily basis. Many people are being helped by their teaching, and we appreciate their efforts very much.

As we mentioned earlier, we have finished writing this book in the early spring. Spring is the time when the vegetable world begins to awaken and produce a boundless variety of food. We hope that this small cookbook, which is like a tiny, compact seed, will sprout and grow into many wonderful and delicious meals for your family and friends. Enjoy in good health!

Aveline Kushi
Wendy Esko
Brookline, Massachusetts
April 1984

Introduction

Cooking is the art of life. Our ability to think and act is a reflection of our state of physical and mental health, which has as its foundation the food we cook and eat. You could say cooking is what separates man from beast, as it developed as an art along with culture. To master the art of cooking—to choose the right kinds of foods, and to combine them properly—is to master the art of life, for the greatness and destiny of all people reflect and are limited by the quality of their daily food.

It is vitally important that you learn how to prepare food that is harmonious with your body as well as with your environment. Just as individual health is built on harmonious living and eating, so is the health and unity of the family. The present decay of the family structure in our society cannot be separated from the kinds of food we eat and the ways they are prepared. It is a well-known fact that highly processed foods, sugared foods, and the chemicals they contain can affect behavior and cause drastic allergic reactions in many people.

The massive change in eating that has taken us from wholesome natural foods to packaged, processed, refined items has caused an equally massive decline in the health of society. Yet, a return to family-oriented cooking and community living can bring health to the individual, unity and love to the family, and peace and brotherhood to society.

The Changing Seasons Macrobiotic Cookbook is different from most cookbooks in its approach to cooking. The foods used are wholesome, all natural, and delicious, and the meals and cooking methods used to prepare them are presented in harmony with the seasons. For just as nature and our levels of activity change constantly, so should our food and methods of preparing it change in accordance with our needs. You probably practice this intuitive approach to some degree now. For example, by serving lighter food and using less cooking during the summer, or by purchasing and eating locally grown produce in season. By being conscious of the changes in nature and in your body, you can adapt to them, and realize the highest possible physical health and spirit.

My wife, Aveline, is an expert macrobiotic and natural-foods cook. The recipes in this book are the result of hundreds of hours of practicing and teaching the art of macrobiotic and traditional natural-foods cooking. Having raised a family of five children without sickness, without quarrel, and without separation, we can attest to the value and importance of proper eating and cooking. Wendy Esko, who graciously helped Aveline compile and organize these recipes, is also a highly qualified macrobiotic instructor with years of experience, and is the mother of five handsome children.

I hope you will embrace the art of macrobiotic cooking through the recipes presented in this book. Simple as they may seem, the changes that macrobiotic cooking and eating can bring about in your health and life are truly profound.

Michio Kushi
Brookline, Massachusetts
September 1984

The Art of Cooking with the Seasons

THE STANDARD MACROBIOTIC DIET

The recipes in this cookbook are based on standard macrobiotic dietary recommendations that can be applied to your own kitchen. Certainly there is no one diet that is suited to every need. Modifications are always necessary, depending on where you are living, the type of climate there, the particular season, and your sex, age, job, personal condition, and level of activity. In the temperate, four-season climate that characterizes most of the United States, an optimum daily diet consists of the following general proportions of foods.

General Proportions, Optimum Daily Diet

The general proportions in the standard macrobiotic diet are based on the traditional dietary patterns that protected our ancestors from many of the degenerative disorders that we suffer from today. The diet also enables us to achieve harmony with changing environmental

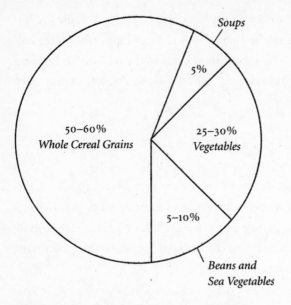

Soups

5%

50–60%
Whole Cereal Grains

25–30%
Vegetables

5–10%

*Beans and
Sea Vegetables*

Plus Beverages, Occasional Supplementary Foods,
Seasonings, and Condiments

conditions. Until recent times, for example, cooked whole cereal grains were eaten as staple foods throughout the world: rice in the Orient; wheat, barley, rye, and oats in Europe and America; buckwheat or kasha in Russia and Central Europe; corn in the Americas; the millet, wheat, and other whole grains in Africa and the Middle East.

In Western countries, bread was the traditional "staff of life," eaten in its whole, natural form until this century. The central place accorded to whole cereal grains in Europe and America is recorded in the prayer with which generations of people have begun each day: "Give us this day our daily bread"—meaning food in general. In Japanese, the term used for a meal is *gohan,* which means rice, indicating the significance of whole cereal grains in the traditional Japanese diet.

Throughout the world, traditional diets have included fresh local vegetables and beans and their products along with whole grains. In many parts of the world, sea vegetables and other products from the oceans, together with a wide range of fermented foods such as naturally aged sauerkraut, pickled vegetables, miso, shoyu, and tempeh, were also traditional. In general, animal proteins, including meat, eggs, and dairy products, were used much less frequently than at present, while people in temperate climates rarely ate fruits and other products imported from the tropics.

Using whole grains, local vegetables, beans, and sea vegetables as our primary foods complements the structure and function of the human digestive system. Our thirty-two adult teeth are better suited for crushing and grinding plant fibers than they are for tearing animal flesh. We have twenty-eight incisors, premolars, and molars, which are best suited for grains, beans, and vegetables, but only four canine teeth, which can be used for tearing animal foods. According to the structure of our teeth, the ideal ratio between vegetable and animal foods is seven to one.

The length of the human digestive tract also favors the consumption of more plant than animal foods. Carnivores generally have relatively short intestines, to prevent the buildup of the harmful bacteria and toxins that accompany the decomposition of animal flesh. Because the human digestive tract is long and convoluted, it is not well suited to the consumption of a large volume of animal protein. The overintake of animal foods often leads to the buildup of harmful bacteria and toxins in the digestive tract and bloodstream, contributing to a variety of disorders.

MODIFYING THE DIET

In addition to eating according to our physical structure and traditional dietary practices, it is important for us to eat in a way that brings our condition into harmony with the environment around us. This can be done by relying primarily on foods that are grown in a climate similar to the one in which we live and by adjusting our selection of foods and cooking methods to accommodate the changing of the seasons.

In general, those who live in cold polar climates may consume a greater volume of animal food, while those in a hot, semitropical or tropical region can rely almost entirely on vegetable quality products. People living in an in-between, or four-season, climate may follow the traditional macrobiotic order in their diets, with cereal grains as the main foods; soup, vegetables, beans, and sea vegetables as secondary foods; fruits, nuts, and seeds as their third food group; and animal foods such as fish and seafood, which are biologically distant from the human species, as the fourth supplement.

If we move to another climatic region, we need to change the types of food that we select and our style of cooking to adapt to the new environment. Similarly, our diet can also be changed to suit fluctuations in temperature, humidity, and other conditions that come about as a result of the changing of the seasons. For example, we can harmonize our diet with the environment as follows:

MODIFICATIONS FOR CLIMATIC FACTORS

	Lower	*Higher*
Temperature	More thorough cooking; stronger seasoning	Shorter cooking times; less seasoning
Humidity	More water in cooking	Less water in cooking

Geographic Range

Sometimes it is best to select foods from the immediate locality, and sometimes you may choose foods brought in from greater distances. The table on the following page provides some guidelines you may use for determining the ideal geographic range for foods imported to your area.

It is better not to import foods across the equator because atmospheric, oceanic, and electromagnetic conditions in the Northern and Southern Hemispheres are opposite to one another. These differences also appear in the food products of each region and result in subtle, but opposite, effects on body and mind.

As mentioned previously, each person needs to eat according to his or her individual condition based on factors such as age, previous dietary history and tradition, activity, racial or cultural background, and physical constitution and condition. These modifications may appear in the types of grains, vegetables, and supplementary foods used, along with the way of cooking and combining food. Thousands of varieties of dishes are possible within the general principles presented above, and just a few of the many varieties of dishes used in macrobiotic cooking are included in this book.

Whole-Cereal Grains

Ideally, at least 50 percent of every macrobiotic meal will consist of cooked whole-cereal grain, prepared in a variety of ways. Whole organic cereal grains that are best for regular daily use include brown rice (short- and medium-grain brown rice), millet, barley (pearl and pearled) corn, whole oats, wheat berries, rye, and buckwheat. Other grains and grain products suitable for occasional use (once or twice a week) include sweet and long-grain brown rice, whole-wheat noodles (udon and somen), buckwheat noodles (soba), unleavened whole-wheat, whole-rye, or other whole-grain breads, rice cakes, cracked wheat, bulghur, steel-cut oats, rolled oats, cornmeal or grits, rye flakes, couscous, seitan, and fu. As you can see, whole grains are preferable to flour products. Flour products tend to be more difficult to digest.

Soups

You may consume approximately 5 percent (one or two cups) of your daily food in the form of miso or shoyu broth. The soup should not taste overly salty. Include a wide range of vegetables, especially wakame sea vegetable, every day. Grain and bean soups may also occasionally be eaten.

FOOD OR BEVERAGE	IDEAL GEOGRAPHICAL RANGE
Water	Immediate environment; ideally from a well or spring near your home.
Fruit	Same climatic and geographical area; for example, the New England area for someone in Massachusetts.
Vegetables	More extended area, but similar to the place in which you live; for example, the Mid-Atlantic or Midwestern states for someone in New England.
Whole Grains and Beans	Further extended areas that share similar geographical and climatic conditions; for example, anywhere in North America for people living in the United States.
Sea Vegetables	Even further extended than the above; generally anywhere within the same climatic belt; for example, people living in North America or Europe may eat sea vegetables from either place or from the temperate zones of the Far East.
Sea Salt	The entire hemisphere, either Northern or Southern, depending upon where you live.

Vegetables

About 25 to 30 percent of each macrobiotic meal may consist of vegetables. Two-thirds of these may be cooked in various styles (sautéed, steamed, boiled, or baked). The remaining third may be eaten uncooked—pressed in sea salt, umeboshi vinegar, or shoyu and water, pickled according to traditional methods, or prepared as raw salad. Enjoy the many kinds of vegetables that are available (green leafy, root, round, and ground vegetables) and learn to appreciate their different tastes, colors, and textures. Please note carefully the three lists below. Unless you live in a tropical climate, avoid the foods of tropical origin (listed in the last column) whenever possible, because they are difficult to balance in the body.

Vegetables

Regular Use	Occasional Use	Avoid or Moderate Use
acorn squash	alfalfa sprouts	asparagus
bok choy	chives	avocado
broccoli	cucumber	bamboo shoots
broccoli rabe	endive	beets
Brussels sprouts	escarole	eggplant
burdock	green peas	ginseng
buttercup squash	green snap (string) beans	green and red peppers
butternut squash	kohlrabi and greens	Jerusalem artichokes
carrot tops	lettuce	okra
carrots	mung bean sprouts	potatoes
cauliflower	mushrooms	spinach
celery	patty pan squash	sweet potatoes
chicory	red cabbage	Swiss chard
Chinese cabbage	rutabaga	taro (large ones)
collard greens	shiitake mushrooms	tomatoes
daikon, fresh or dried	snowpeas	yams
dandelion greens	soybean sprouts	zucchini
fresh corn	summer squashes	
garden or wintercress	taro (small ones)	
ginger	yellow wax beans	
green cabbage		
Hokkaido pumpkin		
Hubbard squash		
kale		
leeks		
lotus root, fresh or dried		
lotus seeds		
mustard greens		
onions		
parsley		
parsnips		
pumpkin		
red radishes and greens		
scallions		
turnip greens		
turnips		
watercress		

Beans and Sea Vegetables

About 5 to 10 percent of your daily diet may consist of cooked beans and sea vegetables. The most suitable beans for regular use are azuki beans, chick peas, and green lentils. Other beans that may be eaten on occasion include kidney beans, split peas, red lentils, navy beans, soybeans, turtle beans, Japanese black soybeans, pinto beans, and lima beans. Delicious bean products such as tempeh, natto, and fresh or dried tofu also may be enjoyed several times per week. Sea vegetables such as hiziki, arame, kombu, wakame, nori, green nori flakes, dulse, agar-agar, and kelp can be prepared in a variety of ways—cooked with beans or vegetables, added to soups, or eaten separately as side dishes—and flavored with a moderate amount of shoyu soy sauce, sea salt, or miso.

Supplementary Foods

This category may make up 5 to 10 percent of the overall food intake. The foods in this category include sweeteners, fruits, nuts, and beverages. They are optional in the sense that in some cases they may be included while in others they may need to be avoided. In general, those in good overall health may enjoy the supplementary items mentioned below. Persons with specific disorders are advised to seek the guidance of experienced macrobiotic friends or counselors regarding modifications of the standard diet.

Once or twice a week, a small amount of white-meat fish may be eaten if you desire and your present condition allows. Fruit desserts, as well as fresh and dried fruits (locally grown fruits only) may also be eaten on occasion. If you live in a temperate zone (most of the continental United States is temperate), avoid tropical and semitropical fruit. The use of fruit juice is not advisable. However, occasionally in warm weather it is all right, provided you are in good health.

Roasted seeds that have been lightly seasoned with tamari soy sauce may be enjoyed as a snack or supplement. These include squash, pumpkin, sunflower, and sesame seeds.

Snacks such as rice cakes, puffed whole cereals, and popcorn may also be enjoyed from time to time, together with low-fat, northern varieties of nuts. Like seeds, nuts may be roasted in a skillet with a little tamari soy sauce.

Beverages. The beverages recommended for daily use include roasted bancha (kukicha) twig tea, roasted brown rice tea, toasted barley tea (mugicha), dandelion tea, and cereal grain coffee. Any traditional tea that does not have an aromatic fragrance or a stimulant effect may be used on the macrobiotic diet.

Sweeteners, Fruits, Seeds, and Nuts

Occasional Use	Very Occasional Use	Avoid or Moderate Use
amazake	almonds	bananas
apple cider	filberts	Brazil nuts
apple juice	lemons	cashews
apples, fresh or dried	peanuts	coconuts
apricots	pecans	dates
barley malt	tangerines	figs
blackberries	walnuts	grapefruits
blueberries		kiwi
cantaloupe		mangoes
cherries		oranges
chestnuts		papayas
dried temperate-climate		pistachios
fruits		tangelos
grapes		
honeydew melon		
peaches		
pears		
plums		
prunes		
pumpkin seeds		
raisins		
raspberries		
rice syrup		
sesame seeds		
squash seeds		
strawberries		
sunflower seeds		
watermelon		

Condiments. It is beneficial to use condiments with your food, particularly with grains. The main condiments used in macrobiotic cooking are umeboshi plum, sea vegetable powders, roasted sesame seeds, sea salt (gomashio), and tekka.

SUGGESTIONS FOR DAILY LIFE

Together with eating well, there are a number of commonsense practices that we recommend for a healthier and more natural way of life. Practices such as keeping physically active and using natural cooking utensils, fabrics, and building materials in the home were once part of most people's daily lives. With each generation, we have gone further and further from our roots in nature, and have experienced a corresponding decline in vitality and a rise in chronic illness. The daily-life suggestions presented below complement a balanced, natural diet and can help to guide you toward more satisfying and harmonious living.

- Eat two to three times per day, making sure food proportions are correct and chewing is thorough. Avoid eating for approximately three hours before sleep. For thirst, in addition to the beverages listed above, an occasional sip of spring water, not iced, is okay.
- Live each day happily, without being preoccupied with your health, and keep mentally and physically active.
- Greet everyone and everything with gratitude, particularly offering thanks before and after each meal.
- Chew your food very well, at least fifty times per mouthful.
- Try to retire before midnight and get up early in the morning.
- Avoid wearing synthetic clothing or woolen articles directly against your skin. Wear cotton garments instead. Avoid excessive metallic accessories on the fingers, wrists, and neck. Keep such ornaments simple and graceful.
- If your strength permits, go outdoors in simple clothing and barefoot if possible. Walk on the grass, beach, or soil up to one-half hour each day.
- Keep every corner of your home in good order—the kitchen, bathroom, bedrooms, and living rooms.
- Maintain an active correspondence, extending your best wishes to parents, children, brothers and sisters, relatives, teachers, and friends.

- Avoid taking long, hot baths or showers unless you have been consuming too much salt or animal food.
- Every morning or every night before retiring, scrub your entire body with a hot, damp towel until your circulation becomes active. If this is not convenient, at least scrub your hands, feet, fingers, and toes.
- Avoid chemically perfumed cosmetics, soaps, and shampoos. Brush your teeth with natural preparations or sea salt.
- Exercise regularly as part of daily life. Exercise includes scrubbing floors, cleaning windows, washing clothes, etc. You may also participate in systematic exercise programs such as yoga, martial arts, aerobics, and sports.
- Avoid using electric cooking devices (ovens, ranges, blenders, food processors, toaster ovens) or microwave ovens. Try to convert to gas or wood-stove cooking at the earliest opportunity.
- Avoid or minimize watching television, especially color TV, as it exposes the body to a great deal of unnatural electromagnetic radiation. Try not to watch TV during meals.
- Include many large green plants in your living room and bedroom to freshen and enrich the oxygen content of your home.

PREPARATION FOR COOKING

Everyone knows that one of the most universal laws of nature is that everything changes. At all times the weather and seasons are changing. Day changes into night and night changes into day. Spring changes into summer, autumn changes into winter. As actors on the stage of life, our roles are also always changing. Our physical and mental conditions are changing constantly. We must at all times be very flexible or we cannot participate fully in the drama of life. The recipes in this book are based on this awareness. There is one full week of menus and recipes for each of the four seasons. These include full breakfast, lunch, and dinner recipes. This will give you a general idea of how to plan your daily menus and adjust your cooking from one season to the next. As many of these recipes require soaking the ingredients and long, slow cooking, advance planning is essential.

If you observe nature, garden, or farm, you will learn what grows in your area and when various grains, beans, and vegetables are planted and harvested. This practical knowledge can then be applied naturally to your cooking, eating, and daily life. Each season has its peak, and during this period different foods, especially garden vegetables, are at their best, tasting most delicious and appearing most beautiful. As you use this book, remember that it is best to choose foods for your daily menus from seasonal foods growing in your local area.

Unlike fresh vegetables, grains, beans, and sea vegetables require no special measures to store or preserve them and can be enjoyed all year long.

Whether you live in a tropical, semitropical, or temperate area, changes in vegetation regularly occur. You can easily adjust your daily menus according to these changes. During each of the four seasons, there is a variety of foods that have a sweet taste. During the spring, for example, the sweet flavor can be provided by snowpeas, fresh local fruits, carrots, daikon, and other sweet vegetables. In the summer, a sweet taste can be brought out with dishes that include sweet corn or with desserts made with fresh local fruits. Autumn offers an abundance of naturally sweet products including squashes, onions, cabbages, carrots, turnips, and others. In winter, we often use chestnuts, azuki beans sweetened with chestnuts and raisins, mochi (pounded sweet rice), dried fruits, squashes, and various root vegetables for a naturally sweet taste. Cereal grains such as rice, millet, and sweet rice are naturally sweet (the more you chew them the sweeter they become), and these, of course, are used throughout the year. The natural sweet tastes can be accented or brought out in various ways by alternating many different cooking methods.

When planning your daily menus, keep the standard diet in mind, and try to include a whole grain, soup, vegetable main dish, bean or bean product, and sea vegetable in the course of each day. Breakfast and lunch are generally simple, while the evening meal is more elaborate and may include many or all of the above-mentioned foods. Also try to include a variety of other tastes within each meal or each day.

By following these basic principles, we can create simple but elegant menus which we can easily adjust with various condiments, pickles, etc.

INGREDIENTS AND BASIC COOKING METHODS

In macrobiotics, we always try to obtain the best-quality natural ingredients. Rather than highly processed, artificial foods, we prefer naturally grown and minimally (if at all) processed items. For example, mineral-rich sea salt and cold-pressed oils are better than refined table salt and chemically processed oils. The quality of the factors used in preparing food is also important. Clean, natural water for rinsing fruits and vegetables, and a natural wood or gas cooking flame are preferable to chemically treated water and electric or microwave stoves or ovens. As much as possible, strive for naturalness in your kitchen.

Whole Foods

It is ideal to purchase organic natural food to prepare your daily meals. If you cannot locate organic food items, try asking your local supermarket or natural-foods store to locate and stock them for you and for others who may be interested. They can locate these much more easily than you might be able to. Try to use whole, unpolished, uncracked, or unmilled grain. When shopping for root vegetables, purchase the entire plant—leaves and roots—whenever you can. Some root vegetables that generally should be used in their whole form are carrots and carrot tops, daikon and daikon greens, turnips and turnip greens, and scallions and scallion roots. The entire vegetable does not necessarily have to be used in the same dish but may be used in the same meal or within the same day.

Salt

Good-quality sea salt is recommended for daily use in cooking. Many people have recently become very concerned about the use of salt. Sea salt that has a high amount of balanced minerals and a lower concentration of sodium is best. A high concentration of minerals in salt does not present as much of a problem as a salt that is high in sodium. If the balance of trace minerals such as zinc, iron, selenium, and magnesium in sea salt is good, your cooking will be healthful and satisfying to those who eat it. You can judge the sea salt quality by tasting it. If the salt has a high concentration of minerals and lower concentration of sodium, it will have a slightly sweet, mildly salty taste. If the concentration of sodium is high and the mineral content is low, the salt will not taste sweet. The taste of food becomes sweeter and is enhanced with good-quality sea salt. Good-quality sea salt is one of the most important factors in influencing how your food tastes and how it affects your health.

Oil

The best-quality oil for sautéing is unrefined dark sesame oil. For deep-frying, light sesame oil is recommended. These oils are of the best quality if they are cold pressed. Occasionally unrefined mustard-seed oil, corn oil, or safflower oil may be used. If you are living in a warm tropical climate, good-quality traditionally made olive oil can be used. A nutritionally good source of whole oil is roasted sesame seeds. You may use these often as a garnish, condiment, or snack.

Water

Refrain from using water that contains chemical agents or that has been distilled. Distilled water is devoid of natural minerals and life-giving force. The best water for our daily cooking and health is well water or fresh spring water. If the water in your area is classified as hard water, it is very high in minerals. If your water is classified as soft, there are relatively few minerals in it. Either of these extremes may cause slight imbalances in your cooking and should be avoided if possible. It is important to have a source of very good quality water available for cooking and drinking.

Fire

The ideal cookstove is fueled by a wood fire. This type of fire is the most natural, and the food cooked on this fire is the best. Of course, wood stoves are not always convenient for everyone, especially in the city. The next-best quality stove is a gas stove. Electric stoves are not recommended. Microwave ovens are also best avoided.

The proper use of fire in your daily cooking is very important. Sometimes we use a high flame, other times a medium or low flame. If you always use a high flame or a low flame, your cooking may be imbalanced. In macrobiotic cooking, the degree of heat or flame used varies with the types of dishes or foods prepared. For instance, if you want vegetables to become very soft, use a low, slow flame. If you want cooked vegetables to be crisp, use a high flame when you are sautéing.

The Clean Kitchen

Cleanliness is very important in macrobiotic cooking. Whole grains, beans, seeds, sea vegetables, and fruits should be washed quickly but thoroughly in cold water before use. Cold water will contract the outer skin or shell of the food and help prevent the loss of nutrients during washing. Foods that have been washed in warm water are often not as tasty as those washed in cold water.

Before washing grains, first sort out any stones or severely damaged grains. Place the grains in a bowl or pot and run cold water over them to cover. Rinse, and pour off the water.

Repeat this procedure and place the grain one handful at a time into a strainer. Rinse under cold water quickly to remove any remaining dust. Your grains will now be clean and ready to be cooked. Sunflower, sesame, and other seeds can be washed in the same manner.

Sea vegetables may have small stones or shells entangled in them. These are usually very easy to spot and can be removed by hand, along with any hard, thick clumps of sea vegetable matter. Most sea vegetables can be washed in the manner described above, and they usually should also be soaked for five to seven minutes or until they are soft enough to slice. However, arame loses much of its taste and nutrients when soaked, so it is therefore simply washed and allowed to sit and absorb the water that remains on it from washing. If you soak sea vegetables for more than 10 minutes, they often become very slippery and difficult to slice, and lose much of their flavor and nutrients.

Most root vegetables and squashes can be cleaned with special natural-bristle vegetable brushes that are available in most natural-food stores. Scrub turnips, carrots, daikon, scallions, and squashes firmly but gently to remove soil. Be careful not to scrub off the skins, however, as these vegetables should not be peeled before use. Onions are an exception—they should first be peeled and then rinsed quickly under cold water. It is also best to peel vegetables (such as cucumbers) that have been waxed. Whenever possible, purchase unwaxed vegetables so that the nutrients in the peel are not sacrificed.

Leafy green vegetables, especially those with crinkled or jagged leaves, can be held under water for several seconds before being rinsed. Watercress sometimes has small snail shells attached to it and needs thorough washing. Wash the entire bunch once or twice and then rinse the sprigs individually or several at a time. When washing Chinese or regular cabbages, detach the leaves from the stem or core and wash them individually.

Beans are first sorted to remove stones and damaged beans, and then rinsed three times to wash off any caked-on soil or dust, before they are soaked prior to cooking.

Organic or naturally grown foods keep fresh longer if they are washed just before use. It is also recommended that vegetables not be cut in advance but rather just before cooking.

Make sure to wash your foods very well, but remember to do so in a quick, orderly, and gentle fashion.

Adjusting Basic Cooking Methods

As we have seen, the standard macrobiotic diet recommends various proportions of grains, beans, soups, vegetables, and sea vegetables. According to our age, sex, activity, location, and season, we must make adjustments in our cooking. The most basic ingredients or methods in our cooking that can be easily adjusted are sea salt, time of cooking, degree of heat, amount of oil, and amount of water.

For instance, if we are cooking for a baby we use virtually no salt, long, slow cooking, lower heat, no oil, and more water. On the other hand, when cooking for an adult, we may use more salt, various degrees of temperature, various lengths of cooking time, more oil, and more or less water depending on the dishes being prepared.

Other adjustments may be made when a person has a swollen or expanded condition, caused from excessive intake of sugars, ice cream, liquid, or fruits. In this case we may wish to use a little more salt, longer cooking time, less oil, and less water than is usual for a person with a balanced condition. For a person with an overly tight or contracted condition from consumption of meat, poultry, eggs, and dairy food, we may want to use less salt, shorter cooking time, a little more oil, and a little more water to correct the condition. Again, we must remember, though, that the body is a whole and no one's condition is totally one-sided. With the guidelines discussed in this section and with practice, you will learn which cooking adjustments are best for you and your family.

VARIETY IN YOUR MENUS

Nature pours forth her bounty with endless variety. The natural splendor is revealed in a variety of colors, textures, smells, sizes, forms, and functions. Our life itself is a continual manifestation of the new within recurring cycles of change. Variety in cooking methods, styles, flavors, types of dishes, garnishes, seasonings, cutting methods, and in other aspects of our diet helps harmonize our daily condition with the varied and changing world around us. Below are a few simple guidelines for achieving variety in your menus.

Tastes

As noted earlier, the majority of our daily food consists of grains, beans, vegetables, and sea vegetables, most of which have a naturally sweet taste. You must also make sure to include the sour, bitter, salty, and pungent tastes in your daily cooking in smaller amounts. This enables you to obtain a wide variety of tastes and contributes to the overall balance of your meals.

Cooking Styles

There are several methods of cooking that can be used in the daily preparation of food. These include pressure cooking, boiling, steaming, sautéing, baking, broiling, roasting, pickling, and deep-frying. Each of these styles or methods of cooking is unique and contributes a different taste, texture, and appearance to the food cooked. They also affect the body both physically and mentally in different ways.

Each of the cooking methods may also be varied by changing the amount of water, time, salt, oil, etc. For instance, beans cooked by boiling a long time on a very low flame are much sweeter and taste more delicious than beans that have been pressure-cooked. And short-time pressure cooking creates a different effect than long-time pressure cooking.

You can sauté with oil or without it. To sauté without oil, simply use water instead. There is also a difference between quick sautéing and long, slow sautéing. Short, quick cooking or long, slow cooking may be used with each of the methods mentioned above.

Colors

Within the vegetable kingdom there are many beautiful vegetables to choose from. Their colors range from greens, browns, and white to yellows, oranges, and reds. If we use an assortment of vegetables in our cooking, we can obtain a wide variety of colors. Of course, we must be careful when combining vegetables to make sure that the colors complement each other and that the dishes we are preparing are very beautiful to the eye. Especially important in our daily preparation of food is the nice soothing color of green vegetables.

Presentation

Depending on the occasion, we can vary the presentation of the food we cook. It is not necessary to have complicated dishes or arrangements of food every day. When cooking for children we must prepare food in a different manner than for an adult. We may need to cut smaller and cook longer so that the food is softer and easier to chew, and very simply but attractively arrange and present food to children. Also, there are many strong-tasting vegetables that children do not like.

To vary the presentation of food, we can sometimes use very small, sensitively cut pieces such as dice, quarters, thin slices, or matchsticks. At other times we may want large chunks or rounds, especially for stews and nishime-style dishes. It is a good idea to familiarize yourself with the many styles of cutting vegetables that are illustrated in this book, so that your vegetable cookery can take on a variety of shapes and textures. In general, chunks are more appropriate in dishes that require a longer cooking time, while smaller cuts are better suited for quickly sautéed dishes or boiled salads. We recommend keeping most breakfasts and lunches light and simple and saving the more elaborate techniques for evening meals. As soon as you feel comfortable with the basic cutting methods, feel free to create new and exciting variations.

In addition, at times you may wish to prepare a kuzu sauce or some other type of sauce to serve over various dishes. This sauce adds a whole different taste, texture, and appearance to a dish. Try to sometimes prepare a certain dish with a sauce and sometimes without a sauce.

Serving Dishes and Trays

A wide variety of wood, ceramic (both glazed and unglazed), and glass bowls is recommended to vary the presentation of your daily food. Try to use different-sized, -shaped, and -colored serving dishes. Serving dishes enhance and beautify food that is prepared. For instance, if you are preparing tofu dressing for a salad or dip, a nice black or dark-colored bowl complements the white color of the tofu. Moreover, if you garnish the tofu with a few sliced scallions, the dish of tofu becomes very beautiful against the black background. If the dish you are preparing is dark, such as hiziki or arame, you may want to serve it in a brightly colored bowl. Also, if you have prepared a small amount of food, it will be much more attractive if you present it in a small bowl rather than in a large bowl that will look three-quarters empty after you have filled it. Yet filling a bowl to the very top is not as attractive as filling it three-quarters full.

It is best to avoid the use of plastic or metal serving bowls, plates, platters, and trays. The main reason for using wooden and unglazed ceramic serving dishes is that they are porous and allow air to filter through freely and heat to escape naturally. This reduces the chance of food spoilage as well as minimizes the collection or buildup of moisture in your food from the condensation of water and vegetable juices. Glass and glazed bowls are not porous and therefore cause these problems with certain foods. For this reason, it is usually recommended that rice and other grains be served in wooden bowls, while dishes containing much liquid or dark juices that will stain wood are placed in ceramic or glass bowls for serving.

Garnishes

Garnishes are very important in creating balance through the stimulation of the five tastes, our sense of smell, and our sense of sight. Much of our appetite is stimulated by the beautiful appearance of food, and we should use a wide range of colors, tastes, and cutting methods when garnishing foods. For example, a beautiful yellow-orange-colored squash soup becomes even more beautiful if it is garnished with a few green and white scallion slices and several small thin strips of green toasted nori. In addition, the sweet-tasting soup will take on a whole different flavor as the pungent scallions and nori stimulate other tastes.

Recommended garnishes include: roasted black or brown sesame seeds, toasted nori strips or squares, shiitake mushroom slices, chopped parsley or sprigs of parsley, sprigs of watercress or celery leaves, grated or matchstick-cut carrots, lemon or orange slices or slivered lemon peel, green nori flakes, dulse flakes, or various sea-vegetable powders, ginger, sprigs of fresh dill, chives, chopped nuts, deep-fried or dry-roasted bread cubes, sunflower seeds, deep-fried tofu strips, thinly sliced kombu strips, and dried fish.

If we use all that nature provides for us, we can create infinite variety and excitement in our cooking whatever the season may be. Garnishes are a very important aspect of macrobiotic cooking.

Some of the recipes in this book call for the use of specific garnishes that we have found to especially complement the particular dish. In others, the garnishes are not included. Experiment and discover which garnishes go well with those dishes. Be creative!

Seasonings

We can also stimulate the different tastes by using a wide variety of seasonings. Each seasoning has a different effect on our physical and mental health. Some seasonings recommended for regular use are: miso (barley, rice, or soybean), shoyu or tamari soy sauce (made with or without wheat), sea salt, umeboshi, and sweet rice, brown rice, or umeboshi vinegar. Good-quality apple-cider vinegar may be used occasionally. Ginger, mustard (including Japanese wasabi—green mustard), mirin (sweet rice cooking wine), barley malt, brown rice syrup, fresh lemon juice, or fresh dill may be used from time to time. Organic maple syrup (as a sweetener) and red pepper (for use in making pickles) are suggested for occasional use.

Seasonings can also be varied and alternated to create balance in our meals. For instance, we may have a very salty traditionally made takuan (daikon) pickle. If simply sliced and served, it is salty and very contracting to the body. However, if we slice this pickle and soak it in a little brown rice vinegar for several hours, it takes on a slight or mild salt taste and has a distinct sour taste as well. Knowing when and how to use all the various seasonings is an art that is learned by experimentation, observation, and practice. We hope that you will study how to properly use these seasonings in your daily cooking to achieve the best possible taste and health.

Cookware and Utensils

It is best to avoid the use of aluminum or plastic-coated nonstick cookware and utensils. In many cultures around the world, unglazed pottery or earthenware was traditionally used in cooking daily food. These materials are still used in many countries around the world. Earthenware is the ideal cookware because it is the most natural. Again, we would like to stress variety in cookware because each type of cookware affects the flavor of the food prepared in it. For this reason we also recommend good-quality cast iron and stainless-steel cookware as well as earthenware. Food prepared in cast iron will taste much different from the same food prepared in earthenware or stainless-steel cookware.

For instance, baked beans taste very delicious when cooked a long time in earthenware, but do not have quite the same flavor when cooked in a stainless-steel pot. Sautéed or kimpira burdock and carrots taste much different when prepared in a cast-iron skillet than when prepared in a stainless-steel skillet. We hope that you will make use of all the recommended types of cookware to create delicious, beautifully prepared meals.

Wooden utensils for cooking such as spoons, forks, chopsticks, spatulas, and pestles are recommended over metal because they are more natural and do not disturb the quality of the food. If your sense of taste is very sensitive you can notice the taste of metal from metal utensils. Porcelain spoons are preferable to metal ones, but wooden ones are the best.

Generally, utensils that are used for cooking can also be used for serving, with some exceptions. If the utensils are burned or stained, they are not as attractive as a nice new wood utensil. In this case it is best to use an unstained or unburned utensil in serving food. With much use, wooden utensils often become discolored. They can be cleaned with a metal scrubber or with fine sandpaper to make their appearance more attractive.

THE WAY OF EATING

It is important that well-prepared natural foods be enjoyed in a calm and orderly manner. Otherwise, much of the care put into your cooking can be wasted. Today, many people have acquired the habit of "eating on the go" or "grabbing a bite to eat." Often, little attention is given to what is being eaten or how it is eaten.

Many people eat while riding in the car or on the subway, while walking or standing, with loud music playing, or while watching television or busying themselves with some other activity. Their food is often secondary to whatever else they happen to be doing at that moment. Naturally, eating in such an unconscious and chaotic manner is not conducive to good health, smooth digestion, or a calm, peaceful, and orderly mind. A few guidelines for enjoying your food in a more relaxed and orderly way are discussed below.

As much as possible, eat only when hungry. Often we find that we may eat even though we are not hungry, simply because it is time to eat. Do not force yourself or other people to eat if you or they are not hungry. It is also best not to overeat. The best thing to do, though it may be difficult at times, is to stop eating when you are 70 to 80 percent full. A very important factor in determining whether you overeat is how well you chew. If you chew very well, especially your grains, you will automatically notice that you cannot overeat.

Most of the problem of losing our balance with our health is caused by overeating. Overeating causes our organs and systems to work harder and longer than they should. This extra work causes the organs to become weak. It also stretches and expands them, contributing to loss of energy as well as to excessive weight gain. If you find that you are overeating, one factor that may be causing this problem is excessive salt intake. You may find that by reducing your salt intake you can easily control your appetite.

The atmosphere of your dining room or dining area should be clean, orderly, and happy. It is ideal if the whole family can enjoy the evening meal together. Lunch and breakfast are often very difficult for the family to share because of busy work or school schedules. Try to spend at least one meal each day, preferably the evening meal because it is a more relaxed time, eating together and enjoying one another's company.

Conversation about the day's happenings should always be pleasant. If you have small children, try to involve them in your evening dinner conversations to make them feel loved and happy. If children feel left out at the table conversations, they will often begin to misbehave or fight in an attempt to take your attention away from someone else and focus it on them. Ask them what they did today or how school was. Dinner should be a cheerful time, not serious and solemn. But at the same time it should not be loud or too emotional.

For proper digestion it is important to sit in a relaxed, straight, but not rigid posture, and have a pleasant attitude. It is best for us to put aside our sorrows and problems and relax and enjoy our food. Anxiety can cause problems with the proper functioning of the digestive system.

Most important, when we eat we must maintain a spirit of thanksgiving. We can have gratitude for the food we are eating, for the people who worked hard to plant and harvest it, for the person or persons who prepared it for us, to Nature who constantly supplies us with everything we need, for our life, and for our family and friends. If possible, give thanks before and after each meal. This may be done silently by yourself or said aloud by a member of your family. If you have children, this type of reflection is a good practice to teach them. They will become very happy and bring much happiness to everyone.

MACROBIOTIC FOODS
AND EQUIPMENT

Some of the foods included in macrobiotic cooking—such as many of the whole grains, beans, and vegetables—are already familiar to most people. Other items, such as the sea vegetables and macrobiotic specialty products, may be new and unfamiliar to the beginning macrobiotic cook. Yet many of these foods have been used in traditional kitchens throughout the world for thousands of years, and are gaining acceptance as their health and benefits become increasingly apparent. For example, most people in North America and Europe were unfamiliar with tofu until recently, but now, thanks to the efforts of macrobiotic friends and a growing awareness of the effects of diet on health, consumption of tofu has doubled since 1979.

Similarly, many people previously unfamiliar with whole foods now use miso, azuki beans, kombu, nori, hiziki, burdock root, umeboshi plums, daikon radish, kuzu, shiitake mushrooms, and similar foods daily and consider them essential items in the kitchen. At the same time, more than ten thousand natural-foods stores throughout North America have made these products accessible to larger numbers of people, and many supermarkets are beginning to carry these foods in response to customer demand. Some of the food items and equipment that we introduce in this book are listed in the glossary.

HOW TO USE THIS BOOK

In this book, we present a full week of menus for each season, with recipes for breakfast, lunch, and dinner. By presenting menus, we hope to give the cook some idea of how to create variety in daily meals, and offer examples of how your cooking can be adjusted to reflect changes in the environment. With a week of menus at your fingertips, you can more clearly see how the preparation of food changes according to the time of day and the time of year.

The menus are only suggestions for use in your cooking. It is best to use them as general guides in meal planning instead of following them rigidly without considering your individual circumstances. If you wish to add or delete certain dishes from a particular menu or change the order in which the menus are served, feel free to do so. For example, you may either prepare pickles several days in advance so that they will be ready for the suggested meal, or begin the pickling process on the day on which the recipe is presented. In fact, any dish in this book may be cooked individually and served with other dishes that you prepare as a part of your own meal plan.

You may also choose to change the ingredients or cooking methods in a particular dish to suit your own needs. However, when adding or substituting ingredients, make sure that the new ingredients are recommended for use in macrobiotic cooking and that they go well with the other foods in the recipe. For instance, if a recipe calls for Chinese cabbage, and you do not have it, you may substitute regular cabbage; or if daikon is called for and not available, red radishes, small white radishes, or turnips may be used instead. When pressure-cooking, be aware of and follow the procedures recommended by the manufacturer of your particular machine.

In many of the recipes, a specific quantity of sea salt, miso, or shoyu and tamari soy sauce is not given. This is because each person has a different tolerance for salt and salty seasoning. One person may wish to have a larger amount while someone else may wish to have very little. Even when amounts are given, it is better for the cook to determine how much seasoning is appropriate in each situation.

Furthermore, dishes that are presented for a particular season—although perhaps most delicious in that season—can, with minor variations in cooking times, ingredients, and amounts of seasoning, be served throughout the year.

Some of the foods used in the recipes, including seitan, tempeh, natural-fruit jellies, whole-grain breads, and sauerkraut, can either be purchased ready-made or can be made at home. Whether you use homemade or store-bought is entirely up to you. When using prepackaged foods, however, take care to select the best-quality natural products.

On the average, the recipes in this book yield enough to serve four or five people. If you are cooking for fewer people, reduce the volume of ingredients accordingly. Increase the amounts when cooking for more people.

As you start to prepare the dishes in this volume, you may find that food is occasionally left over. One of the fundamental precepts of macrobiotics is to waste as little as possible, including leftover food. There are many dishes that can be prepared using leftovers as the main ingredients.

For example, leftover grains can be used in preparing soft-cooked breakfast cereals, whole-grain breads, stuffing for squash or for cabbage rolls, delicious whole-grain soups, rice balls, or sushi, or may be fried with vegetables or other foods to create tasty lunch or dinner dishes. Leftover noodles are good when fried with vegetables or included in soups or salads. Beans can be fried together with grains or used in making soups. If they have not turned sour, leftover vegetables can be used in soups or fried together with grains. Leftover vegetables should be added toward the end of cooking so as not to overcook. In many cases, nothing need be done to your leftovers. They can simply be reheated and eaten along with any new dishes that you prepare.

As you can see, there are many possibilities for using leftovers in macrobiotic cooking.

This section wouldn't be complete without a note on macrobiotic breakfasts. Time and again macrobiotic friends are asked, "But what do you eat for breakfast?" Foods such as miso and other soups, pickles, and lightly cooked vegetables are often not associated with breakfast. In many parts of the world, however, foods such as these are the normal breakfast fare. The modern breakfast of fatty meats such as ham or bacon, cholesterol-rich eggs, white bread with butter or sugared jelly with added chemicals, sugary cereals, sweetened or processed fruit juices, or in some cases, coffee and doughnuts, is not necessarily good for our health. In some cultures, foods such as these are considered just as unusual as the macrobiotic breakfast foods are often considered here. Most people who switch to macrobiotics rapidly become adjusted to more healthful breakfast foods and, in fact, find them quite delicious and appetizing.

Finally, we highly recommend attending macrobiotic cooking classes at one of the many East West and macrobiotic centers in this country and abroad. For your convenience, contact information for the Kushi Institute is presented at the back of the book. Don't hesitate to contact them for more information or to find out if classes or macrobiotic dinners are being given in your area. Cooking classes and contact with other macrobiotic people can be invaluable in helping you to make a smooth transition to a naturally balanced, macrobiotic diet.

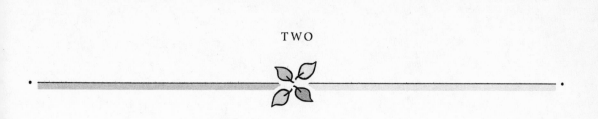

TWO

Spring Cooking

With the beginning of spring, we start to use lighter cooking methods, a little less seasoning, and more fermented foods such as tempeh, natto, and sauerkraut. We also begin to use vegetables with strong rising energy, such as spring wild grasses, sprouts, and leafy greens. It is especially nice to include edible wild plants and grasses from your local area in your spring menus. Wild plants are often stronger than cultivated varieties, and for this reason, it is better to eat them in small amounts. Among the grains, wheat and barley can be included often in your spring menus.

Spring cooking is generally lighter than winter cooking, with a greater emphasis on boiling, steaming, and quick sautéing. As the weather becomes warmer, it is a good idea to eat boiled vegetables or lightly boiled or pressed salads instead of a large volume of fruit. Condiments made with miso, scallions, or chives can also be enjoyed in small amounts. In general, lightly cooked, mildly seasoned vegetable dishes help us to harmonize with the energy of spring.

DAY 1

Soft Rice with Umeboshi

Broccoli and Cauliflower Shoyu Pickles

Bancha Tea or Grain Coffee

Soft Rice with Umeboshi

1 cup brown rice
5 cups water
½-1 umeboshi plum
1 sheet nori
sliced scallions

Wash rice and place in pressure cooker. Add water and umeboshi. Cover pressure cooker, turn flame to medium-low, and bring up to pressure gradually. Place flame deflector under pot when pressure is up. Pressure-cook for 50 minutes. Remove from flame and allow pressure to come down. Remove cover when all pressure is out of the cooker, and place rice in individual serving bowls.

Toast a sheet of nori (see page 121) and cut it into thin strips about 2 inches long and ¼-inch wide. Garnish each bowl with scallion slices and several strips of nori. Serve hot.

Broccoli and Cauliflower Shoyu Pickles

1 cup broccoli florets
1 cup cauliflower florets
½ cup shoyu soy sauce
½ cup water

Place broccoli and cauliflower florets in a pickle press or glass bowl. Mix shoyu soy sauce and water together and pour over broccoli and cauliflower. If using pickle press, apply a little pressure by screwing down the press. If you are using a bowl, simply place a plate on top of the vegetables to hold them submerged in the shoyu-water mixture. Leave vegetables submerged for at least several hours.

The pickles can be left in the shoyu-water mixture for 2 to 3 days and then refrigerated or kept in a cool place for approximately 1 week. The longer the pickles remain in the liquid, the saltier they become. If they become too salty, rinse under cold water or soak for several minutes to draw out excess salt.

Bancha Tea (Kukicha)

1 tablespoon Kukicha twigs
1 quart water

Place twigs in a dry stainless-steel skillet and roast several minutes. Stir constantly to avoid burning them. Place roasted twigs in a teapot. Add water. Place on flame and bring to a boil. Reduce flame to very low and simmer 1–2 minutes for weak tea or 10 minutes for stronger tea. Serve hot.

Grain Coffee

1 teaspoon grain coffee
1 cup water

Prepared grain coffee can be purchased in most natural-foods stores, but if you cannot locate it, you can prepare your own by individually roasting barley, rice, azuki beans, chick peas, burdock, or chicory, etc., and grinding it to a powder. These ingredients can be used in any combination. Bring water to a boil and pour over grain coffee. Stir and drink.

LUNCH MENU

↻

Vegetable Fried Soba Noodles

Grain Coffee
(see page 30)

*V*egetable Fried Soba Noodles

8 cups water
8 ounces (dry) soba noodles
1 cup onions, sliced in half-moons
1 cup carrots, sliced in matchsticks
½ cup celery, sliced thinly on a diagonal
1–2 tablespoons shoya soy sauce
dark sesame oil

Place about 8 cups of water in a pot and bring to a boil. Place dried noodles in the water and stir to prevent lumping. Reduce flame to medium and simmer uncovered. To test for doneness, break a noodle in half and observe the color. If the inside is still white and the outside is light brown, the noodles should be cooked a little longer. When the inside is the same color as the outside, the noodles are done. The entire cooking process takes only a few minutes. When noodles are cooked, place them in a colander or strainer and run cold water over them until they are completely cool. If you do not rinse them, they will stick together as they cool. Rinsing the noodles also helps to remove some of the salt. Allow noodles to drain to remove any excess water (this usually takes 5–7 minutes).

Heat a small amount of dark sesame oil in a skillet. Add onions and sauté 1–2 minutes. Add carrots and celery. Place cooked soba noodles on top of vegetables, cover, and turn flame to low. Cook about 5–7 minutes. Add shoyu soy sauce, replace cover, and cook an additional 1–2 minutes. Remove skillet from flame and mix vegetables and noodles. Place in a serving bowl and serve hot.

DINNER MENU

☙

Rice and Black Beans

Steamed Tempeh and Sauerkraut

Miso Soup with Wakame and Daikon

Boiled Salad with Sauce

Applesauce

Barley Tea

Rice and Black Beans

½ cup black soybeans
2 cups brown rice
2½–3 cups water
2 teaspoons shoyu soy sauce

Place soybeans on a clean, damp towel and rub them gently to remove dust. Do not wash them, as washing will cause their skins to loosen and fall off. Place beans in a dry stainless-steel skillet and roast several minutes, stirring constantly to prevent burning. Some skins will split slightly. When the insides of the beans are a little brown, they are done. Remove them immediately and place in a bowl. Wash rice and place it in a pressure cooker. Mix beans in with rice. Add water and shoyu. Bring to a boil slowly on a medium-low flame, taking 15–20 minutes. Place cover on the pressure cooker and turn flame up to high. When the pressure is up, reduce the flame to medium-low and place a flame deflector under the cooker. Pressure-cook for 50 minutes. Remove cooker from flame when done. Place a chopstick or spoon under the pressure gauge and allow the pressure to come out. When pressure is completely out of the pressure cooker, remove the top. Allow rice to sit in the pot 4–5 minutes to loosen up the rice on the bottom. Remove rice and place in a wooden bowl. Serve.

Steamed Tempeh and Sauerkraut

1 package (8 ounces) tempeh, sliced into
   cubes or thin strips
1 cup sauerkraut (see page 157)
½ cup sauerkraut juice or water

Place tempeh in a saucepan. Place sauerkraut on top of tempeh. Add water or sauerkraut juice. Cover, bring to a boil, and then reduce flame to low. Simmer about 15–20 minutes, checking occasionally to make sure that there is enough water and the tempeh doesn't burn. Remove, place in a serving dish, garnish with a little chopped parsley, and serve.

Miso Soup with Wakame and Daikon

4–5 cups water
⅛ cup wakame, washed and soaked 2–3
   minutes, and sliced

1 cup daikon, cut in thin half-moons
    or rectangles
1½–2 tablespoons puréed miso
sliced scallions

Place water in a pot and bring to a boil. Add wakame and daikon. Cover, reduce flame to low, and simmer for about 5 minutes, until the daikon is soft. Reduce flame to very low and add puréed miso. Mix in miso and simmer 1–2 minutes or so. Place soup in individual serving bowls. Garnish with scallion slices and serve hot.

Boiled Salad with Sauce

2 cups onions, cut in half-moons
1 cup carrots, sliced thinly on a diagonal
1 cup fresh dandelion greens, washed and
    sliced in 1–2 inch lengths

Place a small amount of water in a pot and bring it to a boil. Add onion slices and boil for about 1 minute. Remove and drain, but save the water. Place boiled onions in a bowl. Add carrots to the water you boiled onions in and boil for up to 1 minute. Remove and drain, again reserving the water. Mix carrots with onions. Place dandelion greens in the water and boil 1 minute or so. Remove and drain. Mix greens with carrots and onions.

SAUCE
2 tablespoons shoyu soy sauce
2–3 tablespoons water
¼ teaspoon fresh grated ginger
2 tablespoons roasted sesame seeds

Prepare a sauce by combining shoyu, water, and ginger. Pour sauce over vegetables. Mix roasted sesame seeds in with the vegetables and sauce. Place in a serving bowl and serve.

*A*pplesauce

5–6 apples
pinch of sea salt
water

Peel apples and slice. Place apples and a pinch of sea salt in a pot. Add just enough water to cover the bottom of the pot. Bring to a boil, cover, and reduce flame to low. Simmer until apples are soft. Purée in hand food mill or suribachi. Place applesauce in individual serving dishes and garnish each with 3–5 raisins. Serve.

*B*arley Tea (Mugicha)

1 quart water
1–2 tablespoons unhulled barley, roasted

Place water and barley in a teapot and bring to a boil. Reduce flame to low and simmer 5–7 minutes or until desired strength. Serve hot or at room temperature.

DAY 2

B R E A K F A S T   M E N U

☙

Oatmeal

Onion Butter

Rice Kayu Bread

Bancha Tea or Grain Coffee
(see page 30)

Oatmeal

2 cups rolled oats
¼ cup raisins
5½–6 cups water
pinch of sea salt per cup
  of grain

Place rolled oats in a dry skillet and roast on a low flame for several minutes until oats release a nutty fragrance. Place them in a pot and add water, raisins, and sea salt. Bring to a boil. Cover and reduce flame to low. Simmer for about 20 minutes or so.

Onion Butter

10 medium onions, sliced in thin half-moons (10 cups)
dark sesame oil
pinch of sea salt
water

Heat a small amount of dark sesame oil in a large skillet. Add onions and sauté on a medium-low flame until onions become translucent. Stir occasionally to sauté evenly and to prevent burning. Add a pinch of sea salt and enough water to just cover the top of the onions. Cover and bring to a boil. Reduce flame to low and simmer several hours until onions are dark brown and very sweet. There should not be any liquid left and onions will be almost melted when done. If you occasionally need more water to prevent burning, add when necessary, only in small amounts. When butter is done, allow it to cool before storing in a sealed glass container, or use it right away on your favorite bread, toast, or rice cakes.

Rice Kayu Bread

2 cups whole-wheat flour
⅛–¼ teaspoon sea salt
2 cups softly cooked rice

Mix flour and sea salt together. Add soft rice and make a ball of dough. If rice is soft enough, you do not need to add water to make the dough. If you use plain pressure-cooked rice, add a little water to form the ball of dough. Knead the dough about 350 to 400 times. As you are kneading, occasionally sprinkle a little flour on the dough to prevent it from sticking to the bowl.

Oil a standard medium-sized bread pan with a little sesame oil and sprinkle oiled pan with a little flour. This will prevent the bread from sticking to the pan. Form the dough into a loaf shape and place in floured pan. Lightly press the edges of the dough down to form a rounded loaf effect. With a knife, make a shallow slit in the top center of the dough. Place a clean, damp towel on top to cover it. Place loaf in a warm place such as the oven with the pilot light or inside light bulb on, or near a warm radiator. Let dough sit for about 8–10 hours, occasionally moistening the towel with warm water as it dries out. After the rising period, place the dough in the oven with the temperature set at 200–250° F for about 30 minutes. Increase the temperature to 350° F and continue to bake for about 60–75 minutes longer.

When bread is done, remove from bread pan and place on a rack to cool. Slice and serve.

For variation a few raisins or roasted seeds may be kneaded into the dough at the beginning.

L U N C H   M E N U

Boiled Buckwheat and Vegetables

Bancha Tea
(see page 30)

*B*oiled Buckwheat and Vegetables

4 cups water
2 cups buckwheat groats, washed
1 cup onions, sliced in half-moons
1 cup cabbage, cut in 1–2 inch chunks
½ cup carrots, halved lengthwise and
   sliced on a diagonal
pinch of sea salt per cup of buckwheat groats
1 tablespoon finely chopped parsley

Bring 4 cups of water to a boil. Place the washed buckwheat groats in a dry skillet and dry-roast about 4–5 minutes, stirring constantly to roast evenly and prevent burning. Remove groats and place them in the pot of boiling water. Add onions, cabbage, carrots, and sea salt. Cover and bring to a boil again. Reduce flame to low and simmer approximately 20 minutes. Remove and place in a serving bowl. Fluff up cooked buckwheat and vegetables by gently mixing or tossing. This will allow heat and moisture to escape. Garnish with chopped parsley, and serve.

DINNER MENU

Brown Rice and Wheat Berries

Lentil Soup

Steamed Kale and Carrots

Whole Onions and Miso with Parsley

Plum Tarts or Stewed Plums

Brown Rice and Wheat Berries

2 cups brown rice
½ cup wheat berries (red winter variety),
*   soaked 6–8 hours*
3–3½ cups of water
pinch of sea salt per cup of grain

Place washed rice in a pressure cooker. Mix soaked wheat berries in thoroughly. Add water. Do not add salt or cover pressure cooker. Place on a low flame 15–20 minutes. Add salt and place cover on pressure cooker. Turn flame high and bring to pressure. When pressure is up, reduce flame to medium-low and place flame deflector under cooker. Cook for 50 minutes. When rice is done, remove from flame and place a chopstick or spoon under the pressure gauge to allow pressure to escape more quickly. When all pressure is out, remove cover. Let rice sit for 4–5 minutes and then place in a wooden bowl. Garnish with a sprig of parsley or watercress to serve.

Lentil Soup

1 cup green lentils
1 cup onions, diced
1 cup carrots, diced
½ cup celery, diced
¼ cup burdock, diced
4–5 cups water
sea salt to taste
2 tablespoons chopped parsley

Wash lentils. Place onions, carrots, celery, and burdock in a pot. Place lentils on top of the vegetables, add water, and bring to a boil. Reduce flame to medium-low and cover. Simmer approximately 45 minutes. Add sea salt to taste and simmer another 15 minutes or so. Add chopped parsley before serving.

Steamed Kale and Carrots

2 cups fresh kale, washed and sliced
1 cup carrots, washed and sliced
water

Place a small amount of liquid in a pot. Place a folding metal steamer or bamboo steamer in or on the pot. Place carrots in the steamer. Bring water to a boil and cover. Steam carrots but do not allow them to lose their crispness. Remove carrots and place in a bowl. Place kale in steamer and steam until done. Kale should be bright green and slightly crisp, not limp, when cooked. Remove kale and mix with steamed carrots.

Whole Onions and Miso with Parsley

5–6 medium-sized onions, peeled and left whole
2 square inches (measurement after soaking)
  kombu, soaked and sliced
2 cups water (approximately)
1–1½ tablespoons puréed barley miso
2 tablespoons chopped parsley
1½–2 teaspoons kuzu

Makes 6–8 shallow slices in each onion to create a sectional effect. If you slice too deeply, onions will fall apart. Slicing will cause the onions to open slightly while cooking.

Place kombu in the bottom of a pot and set onions on top of it. Add water to half cover the onions. Place several dabs of puréed miso on top of each onion. Cover and bring to a boil. Reduce flame to low and simmer until onions are soft and translucent. Remove onions and place in a serving dish. Pour remaining liquid, about 1½ cups, over the onions. If too much liquid remains in the pot, thicken it with 1½–2 teaspoons kuzu, diluted in a little water. Pour kuzu sauce over the onions. Garnish with chopped parsley and serve.

Plum Tarts

12 plums (5½–6 cups, halved)
1½ cups water
½–¾ cup raisins
pinch of sea salt
3 tablespoons barley malt
3 tablespoons kuzu
⅓ cup chopped walnuts
pastry dough

Wash plums, cut them in half, discard pits, and slice. Place water, raisins, sea salt, barley malt, and plums in a saucepan. Cover and bring to a boil. Reduce flame to low and simmer about 5 minutes. Dilute kuzu with about 6 tablespoons of water and stir until smooth. Add to fruit mixture, stirring constantly to prevent burning. Simmer 1–2 minutes or until kuzu has thickened and become translucent. Mix in nuts. Remove and set aside for a moment.

Prepare a pastry dough as you would for a pie (see page 102). Roll out the dough and cut it to size for the tart shells. If you do not have the proper pans for tarts, you may substitute by lining muffin tins with pastry dough, or by making a plum pie. After lining tart shells with pastry dough, pinch the outside edges of the crust or press down with a fork to make an attractive design around the edges. Prebake the pastry shells in a 375° oven for about 10–12 minutes. Remove and fill shells with plum and raisin mixture. Place in the oven again and bake for another 10–15 minutes or until crust is golden brown. Remove and serve.

For those of you who must for health reasons restrict the use of or eliminate flour products from your diet, the following stewed plums recipe is suitable, as it contains no flour.

Stewed Plums

12 plums, halved (5½–6 cups)
3 cups water
½ cup raisins
pinch of sea salt
¼ cup barley malt
4 tablespoons kuzu
¼ cup slivered almonds, roasted slightly

Wash plums, slice in half, and remove pits. Place water, raisins, sea salt, barley malt, and plums in a saucepan. Bring to a boil. Cover and reduce flame to medium-low. Simmer about 7–10 minutes. Dilute kuzu with about 8 tablespoons of water and add it to fruit mixture, stirring constantly to prevent burning. Simmer until kuzu is translucent. Remove and place in individual serving dishes. Garnish each bowl with several slivered almonds. Serve.

DAY 3

BREAKFAST MENU

♡

Miso Soft Rice

Pickled Daikon or Turnip Greens

Bancha Tea or Grain Coffee
(see page 30)

*M*iso Soft Rice

2 shiitake mushrooms, soaked 7–10 minutes
    in cold water to cover, stems removed,
    and diced
5 cups water
1 cup cooked brown rice (see page 46)
1 cup celery, diced
½–1 teaspoon puréed barley miso
    per cup of grain
¼ cup sliced scallions

Place shiitake and water in a pot. Add rice and celery and bring to a boil. Cover and place a flame deflector under pot. Reduce flame to low and simmer overnight. In the morning, add puréed barley miso to taste and simmer several more minutes. Place in individual serving bowls and garnish each bowl with scallion slices.

If you wish to save time, you can pressure-cook the above ingredients for 30 minutes. Season with miso and simmer several minutes more. Garnish with sliced scallions.

Pickled Daikon or Turnip Greens

1 cup daikon or turnip greens
½ teaspoon sea salt

Slice washed greens very fine and place in a pickle press or bowl. Mix sea salt in well. To tell whether you have enough or too much salt, taste the greens. Adjust the amounts to achieve a mild, comfortable taste. Screw down pickle press, or, if no press is available, place a saucer with a weight, such as a stone or brick, on top to apply pressure. When water rises to the level of the pickle press pressure-plate or to the saucer, release a little of the pressure. Leave in the press or bowl for 3–4 hours or overnight. If pickles are too salty, rinse before serving.

LUNCH MENU

Fried Tofu Sandwiches with Mustard

Grain Coffee
(see page 30)

Fried Tofu Sandwiches with Mustard

dark sesame oil
1 cake fresh tofu (16 ounces), sliced into
*   8 or 10 slices*

shoyu soy sauce
2 tablespoons mustard
8 or 10 slices whole-wheat (page 114),
 sourdough (page 164), or rice kayu
 bread (page 37)
several lettuce leaves

Heat a small amount of dark sesame oil in a skillet. Place tofu slices in skillet. Place a couple of drops of shoyu soy sauce on each slice. Fry on one side 2–3 minutes. Turn slices over, place 1–2 drops of shoyu on this side, and fry for 2–3 minutes. Turn over once again and fry 1 minute more. Remove. Make each sandwich by placing 2 slices of fried tofu side by side on a slice of bread, with a little mustard on top. Place lettuce on and cover with another slice of bread. Slice sandwiches in half, place on a serving plate.

DINNER MENU

Pressure-Cooked Brown Rice

Creamy Barley Soup

Fried Soba (Buckwheat Noodles)

Tempeh Cabbage Rolls

Arame with Onions

Apple-Pear-Raisin Kuzu Sauce

Pressure-Cooked Brown Rice

2 cups brown rice
2½–3 cups water
pinch of sea salt per cup of rice
suggested garnishes, if desired

Wash rice and place in a pressure cooker. Add water. Place cooker on a low flame for 15–20 minutes. Add sea salt and place cover on pressure cooker. Turn flame to high. Bring up to pressure. When pressure is up, place a flame deflector under the cooker and reduce flame to medium-low. Cook for 50 minutes. Remove from flame and release pressure by placing a chopstick or spoon under pressure gauge. When all pressure has been released, remove cover and let rice sit for 4–5 minutes to loosen it from the bottom of the pot. Remove rice and place in a wooden bowl. Garnish with toasted sesame seeds, a sprig of parsley, several lemon slices, a sprig of watercress, carrot flowers, chopped shiso leaves, or any of your favorite macrobiotic garnishes.

Creamy Barley Soup

1 cup barley, soaked 6–8 hours in 6–8
cups of water (depending on how thin
or thick you would like your soup)
2 shiitake mushrooms, soaked and sliced or diced
sea salt
scallions or chives for garnish

Place shiitake, barley, and barley soaking water in a pot. Bring water to a boil, cover, and reduce flame to low. Simmer for 2–2½ hours, until barley becomes very soft and creamy. If you do not have time to simmer this soup for several hours, you can pressure-cook barley for 45–50 minutes together with shiitakes and soaking water. When barley is soft and soup is very creamy, add sea salt to taste. Simmer several minutes longer. Place soup in individual serving bowls and garnish with finely sliced scallions or chopped chives. Serve hot.

Fried Soba (Buckwheat Noodles)

1 package (8 ounces) soba noodles
2 quarts of water
dark sesame oil
1 cup onions, sliced in half-moons
½ cup carrots, cut into matchsticks
½ cup burdock, cut into matchsticks
1 cup of kale, finely sliced on a diagonal
sliced scallions for garnish
shoyu soy sauce, to taste

Place soba in 2 quarts of boiling water and stir to prevent lumping. Reduce flame to medium and simmer, uncovered. To test for doneness, break a noodle in half and observe the color. If the inside is still white and the outside is light brown, the noodles should be cooked a little longer. When the inside is the same color as the outside, the noodles are done. The entire cooking process takes only a few minutes. When noodles are ready, place them in a colander or strainer and run cold water over them until they are completely cool. If you do not rinse them, they will stick together as they cool. Rinsing the noodles also helps to remove some of the salt. Allow noodles to drain 4–5 minutes.

Brush a skillet with a small amount of dark sesame oil and heat it up. Add onions, carrots, and burdock and sauté 2 or 3 minutes. Place noodles on top of vegetables. Cover and place on a low flame for 5–7 minutes. Add kale and a little shoyu to taste. Cover again and cook until kale is bright green and slightly crisp. Add scallion slices and mix. Place fried noodles in a serving dish and serve hot.

Tempeh Cabbage Rolls

5–6 green cabbage or Chinese cabbage leaves
5–6 slices of tempeh, 3 inches by 2 inches
1 tablespoon shoyu soy sauce
¼–½ teaspoon fresh grated ginger

5–6 strips kampyo (dried gourd strips for
    tying), soaked and cut into 8- to 10-
    inch lengths
1–1½ cups water
1–1½ teaspoons kuzu, diluted in
    1 teaspoon water
¼ cup sliced scallions

If you are using Chinese cabbage leaves, remove leaves from stem and place in a small amount of boiling water for 2–3 minutes. If you are using green head cabbage, leaves are often difficult to remove. Simply steam the entire head of cabbage several minutes until leaves can be easily removed. Remove leaves and allow to cool slightly.

Slice tempeh and place in a saucepan. Add water to just cover tempeh. Add a little shoyu soy sauce to provide a mild salt taste. Add about ½ teaspoon grated ginger or 3–4 large slices of fresh ginger. Bring to a boil, cover, and reduce flame to low. Simmer 15–20 minutes. Remove and drain.

Wrap each piece of tempeh up in a cabbage leaf. Tie a strip of kampyo (dried gourd) around each cabbage roll or fasten the cabbage leaf with a toothpick. Place cabbage rolls in the skillet. Add enough water to half cover cabbage rolls. Bring to a boil, cover, and reduce flame to low. Simmer 5–7 minutes if you want the rolls to be slightly crisp and bright green. For a softer texture, cook 10–15 minutes until cabbage rolls are very soft and tender. Cooked a long time, they are very easy to digest.

Remove cabbage rolls and place in a serving dish. Thicken remaining cooking water with diluted kuzu, stirring constantly to prevent lumping. Season with a little grated ginger and shoyu to produce a mild salt taste. Pour this sauce over the cabbage rolls. Garnish with a few scallion slices and serve.

$\mathcal{A}$rame with Onions

1 ounce arame (about 1½–2 cups)
dark sesame oil
1–1½ cups onions, sliced in half-moons

shoyu soy sauce
2–3 tablespoons sunflower seeds

Wash arame and sort out any stones or shells. Drain in a strainer or colander. Do not soak this sea vegetable. The taste is much better if it is not soaked.

Brush a small amount of dark sesame oil in the bottom of a skillet and heat up. Add onions and sauté 2–3 minutes. Place arame on top of onions. Add water to just cover onions. Bring to a boil, reduce flame to low, and add a small amount of shoyu. Cover and simmer about 20–25 minutes. Add a little more shoyu to obtain a mild salt taste. Simmer until almost all liquid is gone.

Wash sunflower seeds and roast in a dry skillet until golden brown. Remove and chop very fine. Mix chopped seeds in with the arame and onions and place in a serving dish. Serve.

Apple-Pear-Raisin Kuzu Sauce

2 medium apples
2 medium pears
½ cup raisins
pinch of sea salt
4–5 cups water
5–6 tablespoons kuzu
4–5 lemon slices, for garnish

Wash apples and pears and slice. You may leave skins on if fruit is not waxed or sprayed. Place raisins, sea salt, and water in a pot. Bring to a boil. Cover and reduce flame to medium-low. Simmer about 7–10 minutes. Add apples and pears. Cover and simmer until fruit is soft. Dilute kuzu in ¼ cup water and stir until smooth. Reduce flame to low and add diluted kuzu. Stir constantly to prevent lumping. Simmer 2–3 minutes or until kuzu has thickened. Place in individual serving bowls and garnish each bowl with a half slice of lemon. Serve.

DAY 4

BREAKFAST MENU

Toasted Mochi

Grated Daikon with Nori Strips

Bancha Tea or Grain Coffee

(see page 30)

Toasted Mochi

5–6 slices of mochi, 3 inches by 2 inches

Place sliced mochi in a skillet on a low flame. Cover skillet. Toast mochi on one side until golden brown. Turn over and toast until the squares puff up. Make sure to keep flame low so as not to burn the mochi. The mochi is usually done after 3–5 minutes of roasting on each side. Instead of roasting, you may place mochi on a cookie sheet under the broiler for 1–2 minutes. Then turn over and broil other side until it puffs up. Serve with grated daikon and strips of toasted nori.

Grated Daikon with Nori Strips

1 piece daikon root, 4–6 inches long
    (½ cup freshly grated daikon)

1 sheet nori, toasted (see page 121)
shoyu soy sauce

Grate daikon. Cut toasted nori with a knife or pair of scissors into strips 2 inches long. Place 1 tablespoon of grated daikon on each serving plate. Place 1 or 2 drops of shoyu on each spoonful of daikon. Garnish with several strips of toasted nori. Serve with mochi.

L U N C H   M E N U

*Peanut Butter and Apple Cider
Jelly Sandwiches*

Dill Pickles

Bancha Tea
(see page 30)

Peanut Butter and Apple Cider Jelly Sandwiches

8 or 10 slices sourdough (page 164),
    whole-wheat (page 114), or rice kayu
    bread (page 37)
organic peanut butter
apple cider jelly (or your favorite jelly or
    fruit butter)

Very thinly spread your favorite natural peanut butter on 4 or 5 slices of bread. Thinly spread apple cider jelly on the remaining 4 or 5 slices of bread. Place bread slices together to make 4 or 5 sandwiches. Slice each sandwich in half and serve on an attractive serving plate.

Dill Pickles

¼–⅓ cup sea salt
8–10 cups water
1 cup onions, sliced in thick half-moons
1–2 sprigs fresh or dried dill
1 cup carrots, sliced thinly on a diagonal
2 pounds fresh pickling cucumbers,
   quartered lengthwise

Place sea salt in a pot, add water, and mix. Bring to a boil. Reduce flame to medium and simmer about 5 minutes or until salt has dissolved. Remove from flame and allow to cool.

Place onions in a large (1 gallon) glass jar or crock and add about one quarter of the dill. Then place carrot slices on top of onions. Next add a little more dill. Finally, place the cucumber spears in jar or crock and add remaining dill. Pour cool salt water over the vegetables. (If you use hot water, the vegetables will not pickle properly and may become soft and mushy.) Cover the top of the jar with a piece of cheesecloth so that air can get at it. Let vegetables sit in salt water for 3–4 days. Pickles ferment better if kept in a cool (not cold), dark place. When cucumbers change from bright green to a dull green color, cover jar and refrigerate 1–2 days longer. After 1–2 days' refrigeration, pickles are ready to use. In the summer months, when the weather is very hot, these pickles may need to sit out in the open only 1–2 days before being refrigerated. If too salty for your liking, rinse under cold water. Serve in bowl or on pickle tray.

DINNER MENU

☙

Nishime Vegetables

Fried Rice with Wild Vegetables

Clear Soup

Chick Peas with Carrots

Boiled Mustard Greens

Nishime Vegetables

2 square inches kombu, after soaking
5–6 shiitake mushrooms, soaked, stems
removed, and quartered
2 cups daikon, sliced into ½-inch-thick
rounds
shoyu soy sauce

Place kombu in the bottom of a pot. Add shiitake mushrooms. Set daikon on top of kombu and shiitake. Add water to half cover daikon. Bring to a boil, reduce flame to low, and simmer 30–55 minutes or until daikon is translucent and very soft and tender. Add a little shoyu and cook several minutes longer. If this dish is cooked a long time over a low flame, it becomes very sweet. Mix vegetables and place in a serving dish with the liquid. If there is a lot of liquid left, you can thicken it with a little diluted kuzu and pour the hot sauce over the daikon. Garnish with chopped chives or parsley. Serve.

$\mathcal{F}$ried Rice with Wild Vegetables

dark sesame oil
4 cups cooked brown rice
shoyu soy sauce
2 tablespoons roasted sesame seeds
½ cup chives, chopped very fine
½ cup dandelion leaves and stems,
  chopped very fine
½ cup chickweed, chopped very fine

Heat a small amount of oil in a skillet. Add rice. If rice is very dry, you may add a few drops of water. Sprinkle a little shoyu on the rice and cover. Place flame on low and cook until rice is warm. Stir occasionally to cook evenly, turn flame up to medium and mix roasted sesame seeds in with the rice. At the very end of cooking mix the finely chopped wild vegetables in with the rice. Add more shoyu to taste. Cover and cook for a couple of minutes. Remove and place in a serving bowl. Serve.

Clear Soup

1 strip kombu, 6–8 inches long, soaked
½ cup kombu soaking water
4–5 cups water
½ cup carrots, cut in flower shapes
2 cups cubed tofu
4–5 sprigs of watercress
sea salt to taste

Place kombu, kombu soaking water, and additional water in a pot. Bring to a boil. Reduce flame to medium-low, add carrot flowers, and cover. Simmer several minutes or until carrots are soft. Remove kombu and save for use in other dishes or for other soup stock. Place cubed tofu in water and simmer 1–2 minutes. Add a pinch of sea salt to taste and simmer 1–2 minutes longer. Place a sprig of watercress in each individual's serving bowl. Just before serving, pour soup into bowls, making sure to include a couple of carrot flowers and 3–4 pieces of tofu in each portion. The hot broth will cook the watercress sufficiently by the time it is eaten.

Chick Peas with Carrots

1 cup chick peas, soaked 6–8 hours
1 cup onions, diced
1 cup carrots, diced
sea salt
3 cups water

Place chick peas in a pressure cooker. Add water. Cover and bring chick peas to pressure. Pressure-cook for 15–20 minutes. Release pressure. Remove cover when all pressure has been released. Add onions and carrots. Bring to a boil. Cover with lid from pot (not top of pressure cooker), and reduce flame to medium-low. Simmer for 1½–2 hours. Add sea salt (approximately ¼–½ teaspoon) and cook until chick peas are very well done but not mush and until most of the liquid has evaporated. Place in a serving dish and serve.

Boiled Mustard Greens

4 cups of mustard greens, sliced

Place quarter-inch of water in a pot and bring to a boil. Drop in mustard greens and cook several minutes until done. Mix often to cook greens evenly, making sure to bring greens from the bottom of the pot up to the top. When done, the greens should be bright green and slightly crisp.

Place mustard greens in a serving dish.

DAY 5

BREAKFAST MENU

❧

Miso Soup with Wakame and Onions

Toasted Bread with Apple Butter

Steamed Broccoli

Bancha Tea or Grain Coffee
(see page 30)

Miso Soup with Wakame and Onions

4–5 cups water
⅛ cup wakame, washed, soaked, and sliced
2 cups onions, sliced in half-moons
¼–½ teaspoon puréed barley miso per
   cup of liquid
¼ cup sliced scallions

Place water in a pot and bring to a boil. Add wakame and onions. Reduce flame to low and simmer until onions are soft and translucent. Reduce flame to very low and add a small amount of puréed barley miso to make a mild salt taste. Simmer the soup on a very low flame for 3–4 minutes. Place in individual serving bowls and garnish with a few scallion slices.

Toasted Bread with Apple Butter

4–5 slices sourdough bread
Apple Butter

When shopping for a natural whole-grain bread, select varieties that are unyeasted and do not contain molasses, honey, sugar, dairy products, or additives. The best-quality natural breads contain only flour made from organically grown grains, high-quality sea salt, natural starter, and well water. Check your local natural-foods store to find the best-quality brand, or bake your own Rice Kayu Bread (page 37), Whole-Wheat Bread (page 114), or Sourdough Bread (page 164). Serve several slices of toast with Onion Butter (page 37) or any other macrobiotic spread you desire.

Steamed Broccoli

2 cups broccoli florets
water

Place a small amount of water in a steamer. Bring to a boil. Add broccoli and steam 2–3 minutes.

LUNCH MENU

Rice Balls with Umeboshi

Boiled Vegetable Salad

Grain Coffee

(see page 30)

Rice Balls with Umeboshi

2–3 sheets nori, toasted (see page 121)
4–5 cups cooked brown rice
  (see page 46)
2 umeboshi plums

Cut each sheet of nori into quarters to obtain 16 to 20 equal-sized squares. Wet your hands very slightly with cold water. Place 1 cup of rice in your hand and pack it together (like a snowball) or form it into a triangle by cupping your hands into a "V" shape and pressing from the sides and top. Press your finger into the center of the rice ball and insert ¼ umeboshi plum into the hole. Reshape the ball to cover the hole. Then cover one-half of the rice ball with a toasted nori square, pressing it so that it sticks firmly. Press another square of toasted nori on the other half of the rice ball to attach firmly. The rice ball should now be completely covered with toasted nori.

You may need to wet your hands occasionally to prevent rice from sticking to your hands, but it is best to use as little water as possible. Excess water on your hands will detract from the taste and appearance of the rice balls. If there are any spots that are not completely covered with nori, you can patch them up by tearing off small pieces or strips of nori and simply pressing them on as described above, until all rice is completely covered.

Repeat the above process until all the rice has been formed into balls. The proportions listed above yield 4–5 rice balls. Serve them on a plate or tray.

Boiled Vegetable Salad

1 cup cold water
pinch of sea salt
½ cup onions, sliced
2 cups carrots, sliced into matchsticks
1 cup kale, chopped
1 tablespoon toasted sesame seeds

Place water and sea salt in a saucepan and bring to a boil. Add onions and boil about 1 minute. Remove and drain (reserving the cooking water). Add carrots to the water you boiled the onions in and boil about 1 minute. Remove, drain. Boil kale separately, 2 minutes. Mix carrots, onions, and kale together. Sprinkle toasted sesame seeds on top of vegetables and serve.

D I N N E R   M E N U

Millet with Almonds

Baked Tofu with Miso Sauce

Carrot Soup

Chinese Cabbage with
Shoyu Lemon Sauce

Macro-Jacks

Millet with Almonds

1 cup millet
½ cup shelled whole almonds
3 cups water
pinch of sea salt

Wash millet very well and place it in a saucepan. Place almonds in a saucepan. Add just enough water to cover almonds. Bring to a boil, reduce flame to low, and simmer 2–3 minutes.

Remove almonds from water and allow to cool slightly. Remove skins from almonds and add almonds to millet. Add water. Add a pinch of sea salt cover and bring to a boil. Reduce flame to medium-low and boil for 30–35 minutes. Remove from flame. Remove millet and serve in a wooden bowl.

Baked Tofu with Miso Sauce

1 tablespoon barley miso
2–3 teaspoons fresh squeezed lemon juice
¼–⅓ cup water (or enough to make a
*   creamy sauce consistency)*
1 cake (16 ounces) tofu, sliced into several
*   ½-inch by 3-inch slices*
1 tablespoon roasted and chopped sesame seeds
¼ cup sliced scallions or chopped chives

Place miso and lemon juice in a suribachi and purée. Add water and purée until sauce is smooth and creamy. Place tofu in a shallow baking dish, leaning the slices against each other so that they are slightly tilted.

Spoon sauce over tofu to create a line of sauce down the center of each slice. About one inch on each side of the tofu slices should be left uncovered with sauce.

Bake in a 350° F oven for about 15–20 minutes. Remove baking dish and sprinkle a few sesame seeds and a few scallions or chives on top of miso sauce. Place in oven again and bake 2 minutes. Remove and serve hot.

Carrot Soup

3–4 carrots, diced
5 cups water
sea salt
1 cup onions, finely chopped
chopped parsley

1 sheet nori, toasted (see page 121),
    and cut into 2-inch long by ¼-inch
    wide strips

Place carrots and 2½ cups of water in a pot. Add a pinch of sea salt. Bring to a boil. Reduce flame to low, cover, and simmer until carrots are soft. Remove from flame and purée carrots in a food mill. Place puréed carrots back in pot and add remaining water and onions. Bring to a boil. Reduce flame to low and cover. Simmer until onions are soft and translucent. Season with sea salt to taste. Simmer 5–10 minutes longer. Place carrot soup in individual serving bowls. Garnish each bowl with a few strips of toasted nori and parsley. Serve hot.

Chinese Cabbage with Shoyu-Lemon Sauce

2–3 cups water
4 cups Chinese cabbage, sliced on a diagonal
2–3 teaspoons fresh-squeezed lemon juice
2–3 tablespoons shoyu soy sauce

Place about ½ inch of water in a pot and bring to a boil. Add Chinese cabbage. Cover and simmer 1–2 minutes, stirring occasionally to cook evenly until cabbage is bright green and slightly crisp. Remove, drain, and place cabbage in a serving dish.

Combine 2–3 teaspoons lemon juice, ½ cup of water, and 2–3 tablespoons of shoyu. Serve with Chinese cabbage and pour a teaspoon or so over it before eating.

Macro-Jacks

1 cup popcorn
sea salt
½ cup barley malt
½ cup brown-rice syrup
2 cups shelled roasted peanuts

Pop popcorn and season lightly with sea salt. Place barley malt and rice syrup in a saucepan and bring to a boil. Reduce flame to low and simmer 3–4 minutes. Pour hot sweetener over popcorn and mix in well. Add peanuts and mix again. Place sweetened popcorn on an unoiled cookie sheet, making sure not to spread popcorn too thick on the sheet or it will not heat up properly. Bake at 350° F for about 10 minutes or until the syrup becomes darker and starts to bubble. Remove popcorn from the oven and allow it to cool. Baking causes the sweetener to harden on the popcorn. Place cooled Macro-Jacks in a bowl and serve.

DAY 6

B R E A K F A S T   M E N U

Creamy Rice with Kamut

Steamed Tempeh, Sauerkraut and Cabbage

Bancha Tea or Grain Coffee
(see page 30)

Creamy Rice with Kamut

1 cup brown rice
½ cup kamut, washed

7½ cups water
pinch of sea salt per cup of grain
suggested garnish, if desired

Wash rice and place in a pot. Add kamut. Add water, and sea salt. Turn flame very low and simmer overnight. If you do not have time to do this, you can place all ingredients in a pressure cooker and cook for about 50 minutes. Garnish with a few scallion slices or chives. Serve hot.

Steamed Tempeh, Sauerkraut, and Cabbage

1 package (8 ounces) tempeh, sliced into
cubes or thin strips
½ cup sauerkraut (see page 157)
2 cups cabbage, chopped
½ cup sauerkraut juice or water
suggested garnish, if desired

Place tempeh in a saucepan. Place sauerkraut and cabbage on top of tempeh. Add water or sauerkraut juice. Cover, bring to a boil, and then reduce flame to low. Simmer for about 15–20 minutes, checking occasionally to make sure that there is enough water and the tempeh doesn't burn. Remove, place in a serving dish, garnish with a little chopped parsley, and serve.

LUNCH MENU

☙

Deep-Fried Millet Croquettes

Grated Daikon

Boiled Watercress

Bancha Tea
(see page 30)

*D*eep-Fried Millet Croquettes

4–5 cups cooked millet (see page 159)
light sesame oil

In a saucepan or pot suitable for frying, heat about 2 inches of oil until very hot but not smoking. Place about 1 cup of millet in your hands and form it into a firmly packed ball. If you do not pack the millet balls firmly enough, they may fall apart while frying. If necessary, wet your hands slightly to keep the grain from sticking to them. The oil will spatter, however, if there is too much water on the croquettes. Pack the millet into 4–5 balls.

Place millet balls in hot oil and deep-fry until golden brown, turning them occasionally to fry evenly. As the temperature of the oil is lowered with each additional croquette, the balls may fall apart if you overcrowd the pot. You may only have room to fry 2–3 croquettes at a time. Place fried croquettes on a paper towel to drain while you are frying the others. Repeat until all croquettes are deep-fried.

Place drained croquettes on a plate or in a basket that has been lined with paper napkins to absorb any excess oil. Serve each croquette with Grated Daikon (see below) and a drop or two of shoyu soy sauce.

Grated Daikon

1 piece daikon root, 4–6 inches long
(½ cup grated)
1 daikon leaf, 1½ inches long
shoyu soy sauce

Grate daikon and place in a bowl. Garnish with daikon leaf. Serve each person 1–2 tablespoons of grated daikon with 1–2 drops of shoyu soy sauce. When eaten with millet croquettes, grated daikon will help you to digest the oil.

Boiled Watercress

2 bunches fresh watercress, washed
(about 4 cups)
2–3 cups water

Place 2–3 cups of water in a pot and bring to a boil. Drop one quarter of the watercress in the boiling water for about 45 seconds. Move it around with a pair of chopsticks to cook evenly. Remove, drain, and spread watercress out on a plate to cool. Continue cooking remaining watercress in the same manner. Place cooled watercress in a serving dish as is, or slice into 2-inch lengths and serve.

ॺ

Brown Rice with Shiso Leaves

Azuki Beans with Wheat Berries

Clear Shoyu-Watercress Soup

Kale with Sour Tofu Dressing

*Chinese-Style Vegetables
with Kuzu Sauce*

Baked Stuffed Apples

Brown Rice with Shiso Leaves

2 cups brown rice, washed
2½–3 cups water
pinch of sea salt per cup of grain
⅛ cup shiso leaves, finely minced

Pressure-cook as you would for plain rice (see page 46). Remove cooked rice from the pressure cooker and place in a wooden bowl. Mix the finely minced shiso leaves so that they are evenly distributed through the rice. Serve.

Azuki Beans with Wheat Berries

¼–½ cup wheat berries, washed
    and soaked 6–8 hours
1 cup azuki beans, washed and soaked
    6–8 hours
water
sea salt

Place wheat berries and azuki beans in a pot, with azuki on top. Add enough water to cover wheat berries and about half of the beans. Bring to a boil. Cover, reduce flame to medium-low, and simmer about 1½ hours or until wheat is soft. Add water when necessary as it evaporates and the wheat and beans expand. Season with about ¼ teaspoon sea salt, and simmer about ½ hour longer. Place in a serving bowl and serve hot.

Clear Shoyu-Watercress Soup

1 square inch kombu, after soaking
4 shiitake mushrooms, soaked
4–5 cups water
½ bunch watercress, washed
1 cup bread cubes (2 slices whole-wheat
    or sourdough bread)
light sesame oil (optional)
shoyu soy sauce

Place kombu, shiitake mushrooms, and water in a pot. Bring to a boil. Reduce flame to medium-low, cover, and simmer several minutes. Remove kombu and shiitake and set aside, saving them for use in other dishes. Add a little shoyu to taste.

Place a small amount of water in another pot and bring to a boil. Add watercress, stirring to cook it evenly. Simmer for about 30 seconds. Remove and drain.

Heat a small amount of light sesame oil in a pot or skillet. Deep-fry the bread cubes until golden brown. Remove and drain on paper towels. If you cannot have deep-fried foods because of illness, simply roast the bread cubes in a dry skillet on a low flame until golden brown.

Pour shoyu broth into individual serving bowls and add 2–3 pieces of cooked watercress to each bowl. Garnish each bowl with 3–4 croutons. Serve immediately after placing watercress in the bowls, as the hot broth will cause it to cook more and turn a little yellow.

Kale with Tofu Dressing

3 cups kale, chopped
3 umeboshi plums, pitted
1 cake (16 ounces), tofu, drained
¼ cup sliced scallions
water

Place a small amount of water in a pot and bring to a boil. Cook kale 2 minutes. Remove and drain.

In a suribachi, purée umeboshi to a smooth paste. Add tofu and purée until smooth and creamy. You may also add a little shoyu for a different flavor. Place tofu in a serving dish and garnish with scallion slices or chives. To serve, place a spoonful of tofu dressing on top of each serving of kale.

Chinese-Style Vegetables with Kuzu Sauce

3 shiitake mushrooms, soaked
2½ cups water
1½ tablespoons shoyu soy sauce
¼ teaspoon fresh grated ginger
dark sesame oil
1 cup onions, sliced in thick half-moons
¼ cup burdock, sliced on a diagonal
1 cup carrots, sliced on a diagonal

pinch of sea salt
½ cup daikon, sliced on a diagonal
¼ cup celery, sliced on a diagonal
1 cup bok choy, sliced on a diagonal
3 tablespoons kuzu
2 cups watercress, sliced into pieces
    1 inch long

Place whole shiitake mushrooms in a saucepan. Add approximately 2½ cups water. Bring to a boil. Reduce flame to low, add a small amount of shoyu and grated ginger, and cover saucepan. Simmer until shiitake is soft. Remove them and save the shoyu-ginger-seasoned water. Slice shiitake into thin slices.

Brush a small amount of dark sesame oil in the bottom of a skillet and heat it up. Add onions and sauté 1 minute or so on a high flame, moving food constantly to prevent burning and to cook evenly. Add burdock and then carrots. Add a pinch of sea salt, continuing to move vegetables around as mentioned above. Add daikon and celery, then shiitake. Add bok choy next. Dilute about 3 tablespoons of kuzu in 3 tablespoons of water. Add diluted kuzu to shoyu-ginger water. Bring to a boil, stirring constantly to prevent lumping and burning. Season with a little more shoyu if desired. Pour hot kuzu sauce over sautéed vegetables and mix to coat all vegetables. Add watercress and cook about 30 seconds. Mix and place in a serving dish.

Baked Stuffed Apples

1 teaspoon barley miso
3 tablespoons sesame butter or tahini
¼ cup raisins
⅛ cup chopped walnuts
5–6 whole baking apples
¼–½ cup water or apple juice

Place miso and sesame butter or tahini in a suribachi and grind. Add raisins and walnuts. Mix in well. Wash the apples and remove cores with an apple corer or knife. Place stuffing in the hollowed-out centers of the apples. Place stuffed apples in a baking dish. Pour a small amount of water or apple juice (¼–½ cup) in the baking dish. Bake at about 375° F for 15–20 minutes or so, until soft. Remove and serve.

DAY 7

BREAKFAST MENU

Miso Soup with Wakame, Onions,
and Tofu

Rice Balls

Bancha Tea or Grain Coffee
(see page 30)

*M*iso Soup with Wakame, Onions, and Tofu

4–5 cups water
⅛ cup wakame, washed, soaked,
    and sliced
1 cup onions, sliced on a diagonal
1 cup tofu, sliced into small cubes
¼–½ teaspoon puréed barley miso
    per cup of liquid
sliced scallions

Place water in a pot and bring to a boil. Add wakame and onions. Reduce flame to medium-low, cover, and simmer until onions are soft and translucent. Add tofu and a small amount of puréed barley miso. Reduce flame to very low, cover, and simmer 2–3 minutes longer. Place miso soup in individual serving bowls and garnish each bowl with a few scallion slices.

Rice Balls

3 sheets nori
4–5 cups cooked brown rice
2 umeboshi plums, broken in half
water
pinch of sea salt

Toast nori (see page 121), cut into quarters, and set aside. In a bowl, mix a small amount of water and a pinch of sea salt. Wet your hands with a very small amount of the salt water and place about 1 cup of cooked rice in one hand. Form into a triangular shape by cupping your hands into a "V" and applying pressure to mold the rice. The triangle should be firmly packed. With one finger, press a hole into the center of the rice and insert ¼ umeboshi plum. Then close the hole by packing the triangle firmly again. Place one square of toasted nori on one side of the rice triangle. Pack the rice again so that the nori sticks. Repeat with another square of nori on the other side of the rice triangle. You may occasionally need to wet your hands with a very small amount of salt water to prevent rice and nori from sticking to them. Try to use as little water as possible, especially if you are preparing the rice balls to take on a long trip, as too much water will cause them to spoil quickly. If there are any holes or spaces left uncovered by nori, simply patch them with small pieces torn off a square of nori.

Repeat the above procedure until all ingredients are used up. Place on a plate or platter and serve.

For variation, these triangles can be coated with roasted sesame seeds or even gomashio. You can also wrap them in shiso leaves especially made for such use. Instead of umeboshi, you may place pickled vegetables, scallions, or cooked tempeh or tofu inside. The triangles can also be made from fried rice, millet, or couscous. They can be deep-fried occasionally if your health permits.

Steamed Leftover Rice

4–5 cups leftover cooked brown rice
water

Place about 1 inch of water in the bottom of a pot. Set a steamer basket in the pot. Place rice in steamer, cover, and bring to a boil. Reduce flame to medium-low and steam rice for about 5–7 minutes or until warm. Serve in a wooden bowl.

Sautéed Tofu and Vegetables

dark sesame oil
1 cup onions, sliced into half-moons
1 cup fresh sweet corn, removed from
    the cob
1 cup cabbage, sliced into 1-inch chunks
1 cake (16 ounces) fresh tofu

sea salt or shoyu soy sauce
1 tablespoon sliced scallion for garnish

Heat a small amount of dark sesame oil in a skillet. Add onions and sauté 1–2 minutes. Add corn and cabbage. Crumble tofu and spread it over the vegetables. Sprinkle 1–2 pinches of sea salt on top and cover. Reduce flame to medium-low and cook until vegetables are done and tofu is fluffy, about 5–7 minutes. The vegetables are best if they are slightly crisp. During the last 2–3 minutes of cooking, you may season to taste with a little more sea salt or with a few sprinkles of shoyu. Remove and place in a serving bowl. Garnish with a sprinkling of scallion slices. Serve.

D I N N E R   M E N U

Sesame and Chestnut Ohagi

Clear Broth

Kimpira Burdock, Carrot, and Dried Tofu

Boiled Cauliflower and Broccoli
with Lemon Sauce

Sesame and Chestnut Ohagi

2 cups sweet brown rice
2½ cups water
pinch of sea salt per cup of rice

Wash sweet rice and place in a pressure cooker. Add water. Place on a low flame for 15–20 minutes. Add salt and cover. Bring to pressure and cook the same as for plain pressure-cooked rice (see page 46). When rice is cooked, place it in a heavy wooden bowl and pound it with a heavy wooden pestle or mallet especially made for pounding mochi or ohagi. If a mochi-pounding pestle is not available and you pound a very small amount of sweet rice, you can use the wooden pestle from a suribachi. Pound vigorously but in an orderly fashion for about 15–20 minutes. When you have finished pounding, take about 1 tablespoon of the dough at a time and roll it in or coat it with one or both of the coatings listed below and form into the desired shape. Continue coating and shaping the dough until it is all used up.

Other coatings for ohagi can be made from azuki beans, sweet azuki beans, ground walnuts and tamari or miso, other kinds of nuts, gomashio, etc.

Chestnut Purée

1 cup dried chestnuts
2½ cups water
pinch of sea salt

Wash chestnuts and roast them in a dry skillet on a low flame for several minutes. Stir constantly to prevent burning and to roast chestnuts evenly. Place water, salt, and chestnuts in a pressure cooker and pressure-cook for 35–40 minutes. (Note: These chestnuts do not require peeling. They are already peeled before drying.) Then mash chestnuts into the cooking water, using a pestle, or grind chestnuts and water in a hand food mill until smooth and creamy.

Take about 1 tablespoon of chestnut purée and make a round, flat patty with your hands. In the patty place about 1 teaspoon of ohagi dough and wrap the chestnut purée completely around the ohagi. Form the coated ohagi into rounds, rectangles, or triangles, and arrange them attractively on a platter or serving tray. Repeat until all chestnut purée is used.

Sesame Seed Topping

½ cup sesame seeds
sea salt or shoyu soy sauce

Wash sesame seeds and dry-roast them in a stainless-steel skillet until golden brown. Stir constantly to prevent burning and to roast the seeds evenly. When done, remove immediately and place in a suribachi.

If you wish to season the seeds with sea salt, first roast the sea salt and grind it in a suribachi. Then add the seeds and grind a short time.

If you wish to use shoyu, first grind the sesame seeds almost to the desired consistency, about half crushed, and then season with a little shoyu to taste.

Take about 1 tablespoon of ohagi dough and roll it in the ground sesame seeds until it is completely coated. Form the dough into small balls and arrange on a platter or serving tray.

Clear Broth

5 shiitake mushrooms, soaked and thinly sliced
4–5 cups water
1 cup celery, sliced on a diagonal
2 cups Chinese cabbage, sliced
5–6 teaspoons kuzu
sea salt
¼ cup sliced scallions

Place shiitake and water in a pot. Bring to a boil. Reduce flame to low, cover, and simmer about 10 minutes. Add celery and simmer 2–3 minutes. Add Chinese cabbage and simmer 1–2 minutes. Dilute kuzu in 5–6 teaspoons of water and add to the broth, stirring constantly. When broth has thickened a little, season with sea salt to taste.

Place in individual serving bowls and garnish with scallion slices.

If you wish to include a little seafood in this soup, shrimp can be added at the same time you add the vegetables.

Kimpira Burdock, Carrot, and Dried Tofu

1 cup dried tofu
dark sesame oil (optional)
1 cup burdock, shaved or cut into
*   matchsticks*
2 cups carrots, cut into matchsticks
water
shoyu soy sauce

Place dried tofu in warm or hot water and soak for 3–4 minutes. Rinse in cold water. Remove and squeeze out water. Slice tofu into rectangles.

If you wish to cook with oil, heat a small amount of dark sesame oil in a skillet. Sauté burdock for 2–3 minutes. Add carrots and dried tofu and sauté 2–3 minutes. The burdock will become softer and turn from almost white to a more tan color. Place a small amount of water in the skillet, covering the vegetables about halfway. Add a small amount of shoyu and bring to a boil. Reduce flame to low, cover, and simmer about ½ hour or until all liquid is gone.

If you wish to avoid using oil, omit sautéing and boil all ingredients instead.

You can use fresh sliced lotus root instead of burdock for this dish to create a different taste. You may also use tempeh or fresh tofu instead of dried tofu. Place in a serving dish and serve.

Boiled Cauliflower and Broccoli with Lemon Sauce

2 cups cauliflower florets
2 cups broccoli florets
½ fresh lemon

Place a very small amount of water in a pot and bring to a boil. Add cauliflower, cover, and boil until soft, but not so soft that it easily falls apart. Remove, saving cooking water, and place in serving bowl. Place broccoli in the cooking water and boil 3–4 minutes or until it becomes bright green. Arrange the vegetables in the serving bowl so that cauliflower is surrounded by a ring of bright green broccoli. Squeeze lemon juice over vegetables.

THREE

Summer Cooking

In summer, we can use a variety of fresh farm produce, including green vegetables, corn, and summer fruits. Raw salads can be enjoyed more frequently than at any other time of the year. During hot, clear weather, we naturally want to use simple cooking methods, such as boiling, steaming, and quick sautéing, and serve dishes that require less time to prepare. Lightly boiled or pressed salads offer a crispy alternative to more well-cooked vegetables. Corn on the cob can be served often during the summer, and is especially delicious with a little umeboshi rubbed on it.

It is better to avoid iced foods and beverages in summer, even when they seem desirable. Some dishes are more refreshing when served chilled, but it is best not to serve them icy cold. Chilled kanten, vegetable aspics made with agar-agar, or chilled tofu garnished with scallions, shoyu, and ginger can be enjoyed on occasion. A small volume of fruit salad, fresh local melons, and fresh cucumbers can also be enjoyed for their cooling properties.

During the summer, sea vegetables can be prepared in salads or in condiments. Grain, bean, noodle, vegetable, and sea vegetable salads can be served often, while sushi is an enjoyable treat in the summer. Salads can be regularly seasoned with umeboshi or brown rice vinegar, finely chopped shiso leaves, and occasionally with apple cider vinegar or a freshly squeezed lemon.

The tremendous availability of fresh produce and other foods in summer offers infinite possibilities for creativity in your cooking.

DAY 1

BREAKFAST MENU

❧

Miso Soup with Wakame and Daikon
(see page 33)

Boiled Tofu with Ginger-Parsley Sauce

Bancha Tea or Grain Coffee
(see page 30)

Boiled Tofu with Ginger-Parsley Sauce

1 cake (16 ounces) tofu, sliced into 5
  pieces about ½ inch thick
1–1½ tablespoons shoyu soy sauce
¼ teaspoon fresh grated ginger
1 tablespoon fresh minced parsley
water

Place about ¼ inch of water in a pot and bring to a boil. Add tofu and cover pot. Reduce flame to low and simmer 1–2 minutes. Remove tofu, drain, and place on individual serving plates. Prepare a sauce by mixing ½ cup of water with a small amount of shoyu and grated ginger. Top each slice of boiled tofu with a teaspoon of sauce and garnish with chopped parsley.

Vegetable Fried Whole-Wheat Spaghetti

Bancha Tea
(see page 30)

*V*egetable Fried Whole-Wheat Spaghetti

*8 ounces (dry weight) whole-wheat
    spaghetti*
2 quarts water
dark sesame oil
1 cup carrots, sliced into matchsticks
1–2 tablespoons shoyu soy sauce
1 cup sliced scallions
1 tablespoon toasted sesame seeds

Boil spaghetti in water until done. To test for doneness, break a piece of spaghetti in half. The inside should be as dark as the outside. Remove, rinse under cold water, and drain. Heat a small amount of oil in a skillet. Add carrots and place spaghetti on top of them. Cover and reduce flame to low. Cook until carrots are almost tender. (In the summer months, it is best if they remain slightly crisp.) Add shoyu soy sauce and sliced scallions. Cover again and heat 2–3 more minutes. Mix cooked spaghetti and vegetables thoroughly and place in a serving dish. Mix toasted sesame seeds throughout, or sprinkle them on top, and serve.

Brown Rice and Spelt

Boiled String Beans and Almonds

Cool Chick Pea Soup

Hiziki Salad with Tofu Dressing

Strawberry Couscous Cake

Brown Rice and Spelt

1 cup spelt
2 cups brown rice
6 cups water
pinch of sea salt per cup of grain
1 sprig fresh parsley, for garnish

Wash rice and spelt and place in a heavy pot along with the water. Add sea salt, cover, turn flame high and bring to a boil. Reduce flame to medium-low. Simmer for 1 hour. Remove from flame and place in a wooden bowl. Garnish with a sprig of fresh parsley.

Boiled String Beans and Almonds

4 cups string beans
1 cup slivered almonds
water

Wash beans and remove hard stems. Slice beans on a diagonal. Place about one-half inch of water in a pot and bring to a boil. Drop beans in and reduce flame to low. Cover and simmer about 5 minutes. Add almonds and simmer about 5 more minutes. Remove and place in a serving bowl. Serve.

Cool Chick Pea Soup

2 cups chick peas
6 cups water from cooking chick peas
1 cup whole-wheat bread cubes (2 slices of bread)
½ cup carrot
½ cup cucumber
¼ cup chives or scallions
shoyu soy sauce

Soak chick peas and pressure-cook as described on page 55. Purée cooked chick peas and cooking water in a hand food mill. Place chick peas in individual serving bowls and allow to cool to room temperature.

Slice whole-wheat bread into cubes. Toast in a dry skillet until golden brown, keeping flame low and stirring constantly to prevent burning. If you wish to use a little oil, you may deep-fry the bread cubes until golden brown instead of dry-toasting them.

Grate carrot coarsely, slice cucumber into matchsticks, and chop chives or scallions. Place vegetables in a small bowl and pour a few drops of shoyu over them to marinate. Let sit for about a half hour or so.

Place approximately 1 tablespoon of marinated vegetables on top of each bowl of chick pea soup. Place toasted or deep-fried bread cubes in each bowl of soup, and serve.

Hiziki Salad with Tofu Dressing

1 ounce hiziki (1½–2 cups soaked)
1 cup carrots, halved lengthwise and
*   sliced on a diagonal*
½ cup celery, sliced on a diagonal
2 umeboshi plums
1 small onion, grated
1 cake (16 ounces) extra firm tofu
2 tablespoons chopped parsley
½ cup water

Soak hiziki 3–5 minutes and slice. Place hiziki and a small amount of water in a pot and bring to a boil. Reduce flame to low, cover, and simmer 30 minutes or so. Remove hiziki and drain. Set aside to cool.

Place a small amount of water in a pot and bring to a boil. Place carrots in water, cover, and simmer 1–2 minutes. The boiled carrots should remain slightly crisp. Remove and drain carrots, reserving the cooking water. Set carrots aside to cool. Place celery in the same water you boiled the carrots in and simmer about 1 minute. Remove celery, drain, and allow to cool. Mix carrots and celery with cooked hiziki, and set aside.

Remove pits and place umeboshi plums in a suribachi. Add grated onion and grind until umeboshi makes a smooth paste. Place tofu and ½ cup water in suribachi with umeboshi paste and grind until smooth and creamy. Remove from suribachi and mix in chopped parsley. Place tofu dressing in a small serving bowl, and garnish with a little parsley in the center.

Place the hiziki and vegetables in a serving bowl. You may place a tablespoon of tofu dressing on each portion of hiziki salad as it is served or you may mix all the dressing with the salad before serving.

Strawberry Couscous Cake

2 cups couscous
2 cups apple juice
1½–2 cups water
pinch of sea salt

Wash couscous and place it in a fine mesh steamer or line the bottom of a steamer with cheesecloth to keep couscous from falling through. Steam, covered, about 5 minutes. Remove and place in a bowl. Fluff up couscous to cool. Bring apple juice, water, and salt to a boil. Boil 1–2 minutes. Pour the hot liquid over the couscous and mix in. Place the mixture in a glass cake pan or baking dish and press it down a little so that it is a little dense and fills about one-half of the pan or dish. Cover and let sit several minutes.

TOPPING
1 cup water
2 cups apple juice
pinch of sea salt
4–5 tablespoons agar-agar flakes (first
*   read directions on package)*
2 cups fresh strawberries, washed, tops
*   removed, and sliced in half*

Place water, juice, sea salt, and flakes in a saucepan and bring to a boil. Reduce flame to low and simmer 2–3 minutes. Add strawberries and remove from flame. Let liquid cool off a little and then pour it over couscous. Place cake in a refrigerator or cool place and let sit until topping jells. When complete, the cake should be firm, covering the bottom half of the pan, and the strawberry topping should be firm, covering the top half of the pan. Slice and serve.

DAY 2

---

*Soft Millet with Green Nori Flakes
Condiment*

Rutabaga-Shoyu Pickles

Bancha Tea or Grain Coffee
(see page 30)

Soft Millet with Green Nori Flakes Condiment

1 cup millet
4 cups water
pinch of sea salt
2 tablespoons green nori flakes

Wash millet and drain. Place millet in a heated skillet. Roast on a low flame several minutes, until it is golden brown and releases a nutty fragrance. Stir constantly to prevent burning. Remove millet and place in a pot. Add water and sea salt. Bring to a boil. Cover, reduce
flame to low, and simmer about 35 minutes or until creamy and well cooked. Place in individual serving bowls, garnish with green nori flakes condiment, and serve.

Rutabaga-Shoyu Pickles

2 cups rutabaga, quartered or cut in
*   eighths and thinly sliced*
water
shoyu soy sauce

Place sliced rutabaga in a pickle press, small ceramic crock, or bowl. Prepare a mixture of half water and half shoyu, enough to cover rutabaga halfway. Put the top on the pickle press and screw down. If using a crock or bowl, place a plate and some kind of weight on top of the rutabaga. Leave 4 hours or overnight. These pickles will keep about 1 week. If they become too salty, simply wash or soak them to remove excess shoyu before serving.

LUNCH MENU

Udon with Cool Broth and Nori Garnish

Grain Coffee
(see page 30)

Udon with Cool Broth and Nori Garnish

8 ounces (dry weight) whole-wheat udon noodles
4–5 cups water for broth
1 strip kombu, 2 inches long, soaked 2–3
*   minutes in 1 cup water*

3 shiitake mushrooms, soaked 7–10 min-
*   utes in cold water to cover, stems*
*   removed, and sliced*
3–4 tablespoons shoyu soy sauce
1 sheet nori, toasted (see page 121), and
*   cut into thin strips 1½ inches long*
*   by ¼ inch wide*
¼ cup scallions, thinly sliced
water

Bring a pot of water to a boil and place the dry noodles in it. Cook until done. Remove, rinse under cold water, and drain. Place kombu and shiitake in a pot with 4–5 cups of cold water. Bring to a boil. Cover, reduce flame to medium-low, and simmer about 10 minutes. Remove kombu and set it aside for use in other dishes. Season broth with shoyu soy sauce, cover, and reduce flame to low. Simmer 5 minutes. Remove from heat and allow to cool at room temperature or in the refrigerator.

Place the noodles in 4 or 5 serving bowls. Pour cool shoyu broth over each individual serving. Garnish each bowl with 2–3 slices of the shiitake mushroom, several strips of toasted nori, and about 1 teaspoon of scallions. Serve.

Long-Grain Brown Rice with Fresh Corn

Japanese Black Soybeans

Miso Soup with Wakame and Daikon
(see page 33)

*Chinese-Style Sautéed Vegetables
with Sauce*

Fresh Watermelon

Long-Grain Brown Rice with Fresh Corn

1 cup fresh sweet corn
2 cups long-grain brown rice
4 cups water
pinch of sea salt per cup of grain

Remove corn from the cob. Wash rice and place in a heavy pot. Add corn, water, and salt, and mix corn in with rice. Bring to a boil. Reduce flame and simmer 1 hour. Serve cooked rice with an attractive garnish.

Japanese Black Soybeans

1 cup Japanese black soybeans
3 cups water
1¼–1½ teaspoons shoyu soy sauce

Place unwashed beans on a clean, damp towel and rub them with towel to clean. If you wash these beans, the skins loosen and fall off. Place beans in a bowl and cover with about 3 cups of cold water. Let beans soak for several hours or overnight. At the end of this time, place beans in a pot along with the soaking water, and bring to a boil. As beans cook, skim off any skins and any gray foam that floats to the surface, and discard. Reduce flame to medium-low and simmer, adding water when necessary as water evaporates and beans expand. When beans have cooked for 2–2½ hours, add shoyu. To mix shoyu with beans, shake the pot up and down gently. Do not mix. Coating the beans with shoyu and bean juice keeps the skins very shiny and black. Cook until almost all remaining liquid is gone. Total cooking time for this dish is about 2½–3 hours. Place beans in a serving bowl and serve.

Chinese-Style Sautéed Vegetables with Sauce

dark sesame oil
2 cups cabbage, sliced
1 cup celery, sliced
½ cup fresh dandelion greens,
    sliced
sea salt
2½–3 tablespoons kuzu
2 cups water

Heat a small amount of dark sesame oil in a skillet. Keep flame high. Add cabbage and sauté 1–2 minutes. Add celery and sauté 1–2 minutes. Stir constantly to sauté evenly and to avoid burning the vegetables. Add dandelion greens and sea salt. Dilute 2½–3 tablespoons of kuzu in approximately 2 cups of water and pour over the vegetables, stirring constantly to prevent lumping and to make the sauce smooth. Simmer for about 1 minute longer. Place in a serving bowl and serve.

*F*resh Watermelon

1 small ripe watermelon

Quarter the watermelon and slice. Arrange slices attractively on a platter or plate. You can also cut melon into cubes or balls and serve in individual dishes. Sometimes a little sea salt sprinkled on top makes the melon taste sweeter and juicier.

DAY 3

BREAKFAST MENU

Soft Rice and Barley

Broiled Tofu

Bancha Tea or Grain Coffee
(see page 30)

Soft Rice and Barley

1 cup brown rice
¼ cup barley, soaked 6–8 hours
6–6½ cups water
pinch of sea salt per cup of grain

Wash rice and place in a pressure cooker. Add barley and water. Add sea salt, cover, and bring to pressure. Turn flame to medium-low and place a flame deflector under the pot when pressure is up. Pressure-cook for 50 minutes. Remove from flame and allow pressure to come down. Remove cover when pressure is completely out. Spoon the soft cereal into individual serving bowls and garnish with a few chopped scallions, a tiny piece of umeboshi, or strips of toasted nori (page 121). This is a creamier dish than the Brown Rice and Spelt on page 81.

Broiled Tofu

5–6 slices of tofu, about ½-inch thick
*   by 2 by 3 inches*
shoyu soy sauce
parsley sprig

Place the tofu slices on a baking sheet. Sprinkle a little shoyu on top of each slice. Turn broiler on and place tofu under it. Broil for 4–5 minutes. Turn tofu slices over and sprinkle a little shoyu on this side. Place under the broiler again for about 4–5 minutes. Remove. Place one slice in each individual serving bowl. Garnish with a sprig of fresh parsley and serve.

Tofu slices can also be served with sauerkraut (page 157). They complement each other very well.

ত

*Sautéed Seitan Slices with Onions
and Mustard*

Corn on the Cob with Umeboshi

Bancha Tea
(see page 30)

Sautéed Seitan Slices with Onions and Mustard

sesame oil
*2–3 cups onions sliced in thick
    half-moons or rings*
*1 pound cooked seitan slices (about
    2 cups; see page 158)*
½ cup seitan-shoyu cooking water
2 tablespoons mustard

Heat a small amount of oil in a skillet. Sauté onions for 3–4 minutes. Place the cooked seitan slices on top of the onions and add the seitan-shoyu cooking water. Add mustard, cover, and bring to a boil. Reduce the flame to low, and simmer 15–20 minutes or until the onions are soft and very sweet. Mix and place in a serving dish. Serve.

Corn on the Cob with Umeboshi

4 cups water
4–5 ears of fresh sweet corn
2 umeboshi plums

Place water in a pot and bring to a boil. Remove the husks from the corn and wash the ears quickly with cold water. Place the sweet corn in the boiling water, cover, and reduce flame to medium-low. Simmer 3–4 minutes. Remove and place on a serving platter or dish. Serve with umeboshi, which can be lightly rubbed on the corn.

DINNER MENU

Buckwheat Salad

Lentils

Clear Soup with Tofu and Watercress

*Baked Summer Squash with
Miso-Ginger Sauce*

Boiled Carrots and Burdock

Cool Amazake Cherry Pudding

Buckwheat Salad

2 cups buckwheat
4 cups boiling water, sauerkraut juice,
    or a combination of them
sea salt
1 cup celery, diced or sliced
¼ cup sliced scallions
½ cup chopped sauerkraut (see page 157)
parsley sprigs
red radish slices

Wash buckwheat and roast it in a dry skillet for several minutes on a low flame. Boil water or water and sauerkraut juice. Add roasted buckwheat to the boiling liquid and add a pinch of sea salt. Cover, reduce flame to low, and simmer about 20 minutes. Remove and place in a large bowl. Fluff with a spoon or chopsticks to cool the buckwheat and to keep it from lumping.

Lightly steam celery for about 1 minute so that it is still slightly crisp. Mix celery, scallions, and sauerkraut in with the buckwheat so that vegetables are evenly distributed throughout the salad. Place in an attractive serving or salad bowl, garnish with sprigs of parsley and a few red radish slices, and serve.

Lentils

1 cup green lentils
3 cups water
¼ teaspoon sea salt
parsley sprigs

Place lentils and water in a pot. Bring to a boil. Reduce flame to medium-low and cover. Simmer about 1 hour. Add sea salt and simmer until most of the liquid has boiled away. Place in a serving bowl and garnish with sprigs of fresh parsley.

Clear Soup with Tofu and Watercress

5 shiitake mushrooms, sliced, soaked 5–7
   minutes in 1 cup water
shoyu
4–5 cups water
1 cup cubed tofu
½ bunch fresh watercress, washed

Place shiitake and water in a pot. Bring to a boil. Reduce flame to medium-low and cover. Simmer 10 minutes. Season the water with a little shoyu and simmer 4–5 minutes. Add tofu cubes and simmer 1–2 minutes more. Place 1 or 2 sprigs of fresh watercress in individual bowls. Pour the hot tofu and soup broth over the watercress in each bowl. (The heat from the hot soup is enough to cook the watercress.) Serve immediately so that watercress remains bright green and crisp.

Baked Summer Squash with Miso-Ginger Sauce

2–3 medium summer squash
dark sesame oil
1 teaspoon miso
¼ teaspoon grated ginger
water
parsley sprigs

Wash summer squash and slice in half lengthwise. Slice off stem area. Using a knife, make shallow diagonal slashes in squash skin. Then make shallow diagonal slices in opposite direction so as to create a crisscross effect on the surface of the skin. Do not cut deeply. Lightly oil skin of summer squash with sesame oil and place on an oiled cookie sheet or in a baking dish. Bake squash for about 20 minutes at 375° F.

Place approximately 1 teaspoon of miso in a suribachi with about ¼ teaspoon of fresh grated ginger. Purée, adding a small amount of water to make a smooth, creamy sauce. Lightly brush miso-ginger sauce on top of squash slices and bake again for about 10–15 minutes. Remove and arrange slices on a platter, garnished with sprigs of parsley. The squash can be sliced into 2–3-inch lengths when it is served.

Boiled Carrots and Burdock

2 cups carrots, cut in large chunks
1 cup burdock, cut in thick diagonals
water

Place carrots and burdock in a saucepan. Add enough water to about half cover. Bring to a boil. Reduce flame to low, cover, and simmer 30–35 minutes or until carrots and burdock are soft and all liquid has evaporated. Place in a serving bowl.

Cool Amazake Cherry Pudding

1 quart fresh amazake
pinch of sea salt
¼–⅓ cup kuzu
⅛–¼ cup water
1 cup cherries, pitted and sliced

Place amazake and a pinch of sea salt in a saucepan. Dilute kuzu with a little water and add to amazake. Bring to a boil, stirring constantly to prevent kuzu from burning and lumping. Once amazake has thickened, simmer 2–3 minutes on a low flame. Mix in cherries. Place servings of pudding in individual serving dishes and set aside to cool. Instead of using individual serving dishes, you may simply place pudding in a bowl and let individuals serve themselves.

DAY 4

Soft Barley with Scallions and Nori Strips

1 cup barley, soaked 6–8 hours
5 cups water (include barley soaking
    water)
pinch of sea salt per cup of grain
sliced scallions
1 sheet nori, toasted (see page 121) and
    cut into strips

Place barley and water in a pressure cooker. Add sea salt and pressure-cook for 50 minutes. Allow the pressure to come down and then remove the cover. If you have time, this cereal is better cooked in a covered pot over a low flame all night. Place cooked barley in individual serving bowls and garnish each bowl with a few scallion slices and a few strips of toasted nori. Serve hot.

Red Radish Pickles

There are two ways to prepare this type of pickle, depending on how much time you have.

Short Method
1 cup sliced radishes
2 umeboshi plums
small amount of sea salt

Place the radishes in a pickle press or bowl. Break the umeboshi apart and add to radishes. Sprinkle on a little sea salt, mix, and press. Leave for 3–4 hours. Remove, rinse, and place on a serving dish and serve.

Long Method
1 package red radishes (6 ounces),
    washed and ends removed
2–3 shiso leaves
5–6 umeboshi plums
1 quart cold water

Place radishes, shiso leaves, and umeboshi in a quart jar. Pour water over radishes to fill the jar. Place jar in a cool place for 2–3 days. When pickles are ready, radishes will be dark pink on the outside and light pink on the inside. Slice thin, rinse, and serve.

Always rinse pickles before eating to remove excess salt.

LUNCH MENU

❧

*Seitan Sandwiches with Lettuce
and Cucumber Slices*

Grain Coffee

(see page 30)

Seitan Sandwiches with Lettuce and Cucumber Slices

*8 or 10 slices whole-wheat (page 114),
sourdough (page 164), or rice kayu
bread (page 37)*
*8 or 10 slices (about 1½ pounds) cooked
seitan (page 158)*
8 or 10 slices cucumber
4 or 5 leaves fresh lettuce

Take 4 or 5 slices of bread and place 2 slices of seitan, 2 slices of cucumber, and 1 leaf of lettuce on each. Place the remaining 4 or 5 slices of bread on top to form sandwiches. Slice each sandwich in half and place on a serving plate. Serve.

Mustard and sauerkraut are also delicious with this sandwich.

DINNER MENU

❧

Boiled Rice

Scrambled Tofu and Corn

Miso Soup with Fu

Sautéed Chinese Cabbage and Snow Peas

Blueberry Pie

Boiled Rice

2 cups brown rice
5 cups water
pinch of sea salt per cup of grain

Wash rice. Place it in a dry skillet, and roast on a low flame for several minutes, stirring constantly to prevent burning. A stainless-steel skillet is best to use as it is light, easily handled, and heats up and cools off quickly. Transfer roasted rice to a pot and add water and sea salt. Bring to a boil, cover, and reduce flame to medium-low. Simmer about 1 hour.

Instead of roasting, you can boil it in approximately 2 cups of water per cup of grain (4 cups water instead of 5 for the above recipe).

When rice is cooked, remove and place in a wooden bowl, garnish, and serve.

Scrambled Tofu and Corn

2 tablespoons water
2 cakes (16 ounces each) fresh tofu,
  crumbled
3 cups fresh sweet corn, removed from cob
sea salt
sliced scallions

Heat 2 tablespoons of water in a pot and add crumbled tofu. Place sweet corn on top of tofu, and sprinkle a little sea salt on top of corn. Cover and cook on a low flame for 3–4 minutes. Short-time cooking is best for this dish. Mix in scallions after tofu has cooled sufficiently; this way, they will not lose their bright green color. Garnish with additional scallion slices and serve.

Miso Soup with Fu

⅛ cup wakame, soaked and sliced
1 cup daikon, cut in rectangles
1 cup dried fu, soaked and sliced
4–5 cups water
2 tablespoons barley miso
sliced scallions

Place wakame, daikon, and fu in a pot. Add water and bring to a boil. Reduce flame to medium-low, cover, and simmer until daikon is soft, about 5 minutes. Reduce flame to very low. Purée miso with 2–3 tablespoons of the liquid from the vegetables or water, and add to the soup. Mix and then simmer 2–3 minutes. Pour soup into individual serving bowls and garnish with a few scallion slices. Serve hot.

Sautéed Chinese Cabbage and Snow Peas

dark sesame oil
2 cups Chinese cabbage, sliced on a
*   diagonal*
pinch of sea salt
1 cup snow peas, stems removed

Heat a small amount of dark sesame oil in a skillet. Place cabbage and sea salt in skillet and sauté 1–2 minutes, stirring constantly to cook evenly. Keep flame high to make vegetables crisper. Add snow peas and sauté 1–2 minutes longer. Place in serving bowl and serve.

Blueberry Pie

1 quart fresh blueberries
2–3 tablespoons water
pinch of sea salt
2–3 tablespoons rice syrup
2½–3 tablespoons kuzu

Wash blueberries and remove any stems or leaves. Place blueberries and water in saucepan. Add a pinch of sea salt and bring to a boil. Reduce flame to low, cover, and simmer about 2–3 minutes. Mix in syrup. Dilute kuzu in 2½–3 tablespoons of water and mix in with the blueberries. Stir well to prevent lumping. Cook a few minutes until thick. Allow to cool slightly before placing in pie shell.

PIE DOUGH
4 cups whole wheat pastry flour
¼ teaspoon sea salt
⅛–¼ cup corn or sesame oil
¾–1 cup cold water

Mix flour and sea salt together. Add oil to the flour and mix it in well by sifting it with your hands. Add water and form flour into a ball of dough. Knead dough for about 2–3 minutes. Let it sit for about 5–10 minutes before rolling it out. Then divide dough in half and roll one part of it out.

Press half the dough into a pie plate to form the bottom crust and then add blueberries. Moisten outside lip of bottom crust with a little water to help seal the two crusts together once top crust is added. Roll out top crust and place on pie. With a wet fork, press edges down to seal the two crusts together. Poke several small holes in top crust with a fork. Place pie in oven and bake at 375°F. for about 35–40 minutes or until crust is golden brown. Allow to cool before slicing.

DAY 5

BREAKFAST MENU

Miso Soup with Wakame, Carrots, and Broccoli

Toasted Mochi
(see page 50)

Grated Daikon with Nori Strips

Bancha Tea or Grain Coffee
(see page 30)

Miso Soup with Wakame, Carrots, and Broccoli

⅛ cup wakame, washed, soaked,
  and sliced
1 cup carrots, sliced on a diagonal
4–5 cups water
puréed barley miso, ½–1 teaspoon per
  cup of liquid
1 cup broccoli florets
sliced scallions

Place wakame and carrots in a pot, add water, and bring to a boil. Reduce flame to medium-low, cover, and simmer until carrots are soft. Reduce flame to very low. Add a small amount of puréed barley miso and mix. Add broccoli, cover and simmer for 2–3 minutes. Place soup in individual serving bowls and garnish each bowl with a few scallion slices. Serve hot.

Grated Daikon with Nori Strips

1 piece daikon root, 4–6 inches long
  (½ cup freshly grated daikon)
shoyu soy sauce
1 sheet nori, toasted (see page 121)

Grate daikon. Cut toasted nori with a knife or pair of scissors into strips 2 inches long. Place 1 tablespoon of grated daikon on each serving plate. Place 1 or 2 drops of shoyu on each spoonful of daikon. Garnish with several strips of toasted nori. Serve with mochi.

Cucumber-Rice Sushi

Bancha Tea
(see page 30)

Cucumber-Rice Sushi

4 sheets nori, toasted (see page 121)
5–6 cups cooked brown rice
1 cucumber
several shiso leaves or a small amount
   of umeboshi paste

Place a sheet of toasted nori shiny side down on a bamboo sushi mat. Wet your hands very slightly. Spread about 1½ cups of cooked brown rice on the sheet of nori so that it evenly covers about three-quarters of the sheet. Leave about 1–1½ inches of nori uncovered at the top of the sheet.

Remove ends of cucumber and discard; remove skin only if cucumber is waxed. Slice cucumber in half lengthwise to obtain several strips that measure the entire length of the cucumber and are ¼–½ inch wide. Approximately 1–1½ inches from the bottom of the sheet of nori, place a row of shiso leaves or a little umeboshi paste across the entire sheet.

Pull up the sushi mat slightly with your fingers and press firmly against the nori and rice. Continue to roll up the sheet, pressing firmly to pack the rice well, until almost all of the nori is rolled up. Very lightly wet the remaining quarter-inch of nori. Now roll up the remaining part of the nori sheet. The water will seal the nori together, preventing the sheet from falling apart. You now have a nori roll.

Wet a very sharp knife and slice nori roll in half. Wetting the knife occasionally, slice each half of the nori roll into 4 equal-sized rounds about 1 inch wide. If you do not use a sharp knife or wet the knife, the nori may tear and cause the roll to fall apart. You should now have eight pieces of sushi. The cucumber should be fairly centered in the sushi. If it is not, you may have placed the vegetables too low or too far up on the sheet of nori before rolling.

Repeat the above procedure with the remaining nori sheets, rice, shiso leaves, and cucumbers until all ingredients are used. Slice all the nori rolls to obtain a total of 28–32 pieces of sushi. Arrange them attractively on a plate or tray and serve. If you wish, you may garnish the sushi with a sprig of parsley or radish slices to make them more attractive.

DINNER MENU

Millet and Sweet Corn

Kidney Beans

Cauliflower Soup

Arame with Tempeh and Onions

Steamed Kale

Fruit Salad

Millet and Sweet Corn

2 cups millet
2 cups fresh sweet corn, removed
from the cob

6 cups of water
pinch of sea salt per cup of grain
powdered green nori flakes

Wash millet and dry-roast in a stainless-steel skillet until it is golden brown and releases a nutty fragrance. Place millet in a saucepan. Mix in sweet corn. Add water and sea salt. Cover and bring to a boil. Reduce the flame and simmer 30–35 minutes. Remove millet and corn mixture and place in a wooden bowl. Garnish with a pinch of powdered green nori flakes.

Kidney Beans

1 square inch kombu, after soaking
1 cup kidney beans, washed and soaked
6–8 hours or overnight
3 cups water (approximately)
⅛–¼ teaspoon sea salt per cup of beans

Soak kombu for 3–4 minutes. Place kombu in the bottom of a heavy pot. Add beans and just enough water to cover and bring to a boil. Reduce flame to low, cover, and simmer for 1½–2 hours. Season with sea salt and continue to cook until beans are very soft and most of the liquid has evaporated. As the beans are cooking, you may need to add a little water occasionally. Serve the beans in a serving bowl when they are done.

Kidney beans are delicious when seasoned with a very small amount of puréed barley miso. You may also add vegetables such as onions, carrots, or celery to these beans while cooking. Fresh sweet corn also goes very well with them.

Cauliflower Soup

1 head cauliflower
4–5 cups water
sea salt
½ cup carrots, cut into flower shapes
chopped parsley
1 sheet nori, toasted (see page 121),
     and cut into strips

Wash cauliflower and cut into chunks. Place cauliflower and water in a pot. Add a pinch of sea salt and bring to a boil on a high flame. Reduce flame to medium-low, cover, and simmer until the cauliflower is very soft. Purée cauliflower and cooking water in a hand food mill and place back in the pot. Parboil carrot flowers in a separate pot. Remove and drain. Season cauliflower soup with a little sea salt and simmer several minutes longer. Pour soup into individual serving bowls and garnish each portion with 2 carrot flowers, a small amount of chopped parsley, and a few strips of toasted nori. Serve.

Arame with Tempeh and Onions

dark sesame oil
1 cup onions, sliced in half-moons
1–1½ cups tempeh, cubed
1 ounce arame (about 1½–2 cups,
     washed and drained)
water
shoyu soy sauce

Heat a little dark sesame oil in a skillet. Add onions and tempeh. Sauté 1–2 minutes or until onions are translucent. Add the arame. Add water to almost cover the tempeh and season with a small amount of shoyu soy sauce. Cover, bring to a boil, and then reduce flame to low. Simmer 40–45 minutes. Add a little more shoyu for a mild taste. Simmer until almost all the remaining liquid is gone.

Steamed Kale

2 cups kale, sliced
water

Place about ½ inch of water in a pot. Place kale in a steamer basket which sets down inside or on top of the pot. Cover, bring to a boil, and steam. The kale should be bright green when done. Place in a serving bowl and serve.

Instead of slicing kale first, 4–5 whole leaves may be steamed or boiled and then sliced when they are done. This way of cooking vegetables, especially greens, is delicious because most of the natural juices and nutrients remain in the vegetables and are not lost when the vegetables are cut and placed in the cooking water.

Fruit Salad

lettuce leaves
½ cup honeydew melon, cubed
½ cup cantaloupe, cubed
½ cup watermelon, shaped in balls with
    a melon ball scoop
½ cup blueberries
pinch of sea salt

Place a few fresh green lettuce leaves in the bottom of a bowl. Mix the fruit and place it in the bowl. Sprinkle with a pinch of sea salt, mix, and allow to sit about 15 minutes or so before placing on top of the lettuce leaves. Serve.

DAY 6

B R E A K F A S T   M E N U

❧

*Buckwheat Pancakes with Apple-Raisin-
Kuzu Sauce*

Chinese Cabbage Pickles

Bancha Tea or Grain Coffee
(see page 30)

*B*uckwheat Pancakes with Apple-Raisin-Kuzu Sauce

1 cup buckwheat flour
½ cup whole-wheat pastry flour
1½ tsp. non-aluminum baking powder
⅛ teaspoon sea salt
1⅓ cups water
light sesame oil

Combine dry ingredients. Add water to create the desired consistency for pancakes. Mix very well with a spoon or whisk. Let the batter sit in a warm place overnight so that it begins to ferment. This will help the pancakes to rise and become lighter.

Oil a pancake griddle or skillet lightly with light sesame oil and heat. Place a small amount of batter to form a round cake. Fry on one side until little air bubbles start to appear on the uncooked side of the pancake. Turn pancake over and fry the other side until golden brown. Be careful not to have flame too high or pancakes will burn.

APPLE-RAISIN-KUZU SAUCE
3 cups apples
½ cup raisins
3–4 cups apple juice
pinch of sea salt
3–4 tablespoons kuzu

Wash apples and peel if non-organic. Slice apples and set aside. Place raisins in juice and bring to a boil. Reduce flame to medium-low. Add a pinch of sea salt. Cover and simmer about 10 minutes. Add apples, cover, and cook until apples are soft. Dilute kuzu in ¼ cup of cold water. Add to apple mixture, stirring constantly to prevent lumping. Simmer until thick. Spoon over pancakes and serve hot.

If the sauce is not sweet enough for you, you may add a small amount of rice syrup or barley malt.

Other kinds of fruit in season, such as pears, cherries, strawberries, blueberries, and peaches can be used instead of apples. You can also use dried fruit instead of fresh, but it must be soaked, chopped, and cooked longer than fresh fruit.

Chinese Cabbage Pickles

There are several ways to make these pickles. Some methods are short and quick, while others require a longer time. Other variations appear elsewhere in this book.

1 head Chinese cabbage
¼ cup sea salt (approximately)

Wash cabbage leaves by individually removing them from the head. Place in a colander or clean dish drainer to allow water to drain. When all water has drained off cabbage leaves, the cabbage is ready to use. Sprinkle a thin layer of sea salt in the bottom of a ceramic crock or wooden keg. Layer whole cabbage leaves and salt in the key or crock, alternating salt and cabbage. The bottom and top layers of the crock or keg should always be salt. Place a layer of leaves aligned in one direction, add a thin layer of salt. Then align a layer of leaves opposite in direction to the first layer. Next add a layer of salt, then another layer of leaves. Several pinches of sea salt are all that is needed between each layer of cabbage leaves. You may also add a whole strip of kombu to the bottom of the crock or keg. The kombu absorbs water, adds minerals, and changes the taste of the pickles.

Place a plate or wood disk on top of the last layer of cabbage and sea salt. Set several heavy, clean rocks or a heavy weight on top of the plate or disk to press the leaves down. If water doesn't start to come out of the cabbage within 10–12 hours, you do not have enough salt. Pickles will spoil if not enough salt is used.

When water rises up to the level of the plate or disk, remove some of the weight so that the level drops just below the plate. Check the water level every day and make sure that all is going well. You may rinse, slice, and eat the pickles after 3–4 days, or leave them several days longer for a more sour taste. Excess salt can be washed off by dipping pickles in cold water or soaking them a short time. Store in a cool, dark place.

If you find that pickles are beginning to spoil, add more salt, more pressure, or skim the mold. If the pickles get very moldy, throw them out or use them in a compost heap and start again. Pickle making is an art that requires time and patience to master, but the results are well worth the investment.

ʊ

*Baked Corn on the Cob with
Ginger-Shoyu Sauce*

Whole-Wheat or Rice Kayu Bread
(see pages 114 and 37)

Onion Butter
(see page 37)

Grain Coffee
(see page 30)

*B*aked Corn-on-the-Cob with Ginger-Shoyu Sauce

4–5 ears fresh sweet corn
½ teaspoon fresh grated ginger
1–2 tablespoons shoyu soy sauce
¼ cup water

Remove thick outer leaves from each ear of corn, leaving inner leaves on. Remove only the long outer brown tassels or silk from the corn. Rinse each ear under cold water to moisten. Place corn in the oven at 350° F and bake for about 20–25 minutes. Place baked corn on the cob in a basket or wooden bowl.

Mix ginger, shoyu soy sauce, and water in a bowl. Pour a teaspoon or so of this sauce over each ear of corn just before eating.

Whole-Wheat Bread

8 cups whole-wheat flour
¼–½ teaspoon sea salt
2 tablespoons sesame oil
    (optional)
spring water

Mix flour and salt, add oil, and sift thoroughly together by hand. Form a ball of dough by adding just enough water and knead 300–350 times. Oil 2 bread pans with sesame oil and place dough in pans. Place damp cloth over pans and let sit for 8–12 hours in a warm place. After dough has risen, bake at 200° F for 15 minutes and then 1¼ hours longer at 350° F.

Dinner Menu

☙

Brown Rice and Lotus Seeds

Dried Tofu, Carrots, and Onions

Whole-Wheat Somen and Broth

Boiled Cabbage

Cherry Strudel

Brown Rice and Lotus Seeds

2 cups brown rice
½ cup lotus seeds, soaked 3–4 hours
2½ cups water
pinch of sea salt per cup of grain

Wash rice and place in a pressure cooker. Add soaked lotus seeds and water. Heat on a low flame for 15–20 minutes. Add sea salt and turn flame to high. Place cover on pressure cooker and bring to pressure. When pressure is up, lower flame to medium-low and place a flame deflector under cooker. Pressure-cook for 50 minutes. When rice is cooked, remove from flame and bring pressure down. When all pressure is out, remove cover. Let rice sit for 4–5 minutes, uncovered, then remove and place in a wooden bowl. Serve.

For a heartier variation of this dish, see page 184.

Dried Tofu, Carrots, and Onions

dark sesame oil
1 cup onions, sliced in half-moons
1 cup dried tofu, soaked and sliced
1 cup carrots, cut into matchsticks
water
shoyu soy sauce

Soak tofu for 10 minutes. Heat a small amount of sesame oil in a skillet. Add onions and sauté 1–2 minutes. Add tofu and sauté 1–2 minutes. Add carrots and enough water to cover bottom of skillet. Bring to a boil. Add a small amount of shoyu soy sauce. Lower flame and cover. Simmer several minutes until the carrots and onions are tender. Season with a little shoyu mix, and sauté until all liquid is gone. Place in a serving bowl and serve.

Whole-Wheat Somen and Broth

1 pound whole-wheat somen
1 strip kombu, 2 inches long, soaked
4–5 cups water
shoyu soy sauce
sliced scallions
toasted nori strips (see page 121)

Place somen in a pot of boiling water and cook until done. Somen are very thin and cook very quickly. To test for doneness, break a noodle in half. The inside should be as dark as the outside.

Prepare the broth in another pot. Bring kombu and 4–5 cups of water to a boil. Reduce flame to medium-low, cover, and simmer several minutes. Remove kombu and set it aside for future use in soups, vegetable dishes, etc. Season water with a little shoyu and simmer several more minutes.

Place individual portions of somen in serving bowls. Pour hot broth over the noodles. Garnish with a few scallion slices and toasted nori strips. Serve hot.

Boiled Cabbage

3 cups cabbage, sliced
chopped parsley
water

Boil a small amount of water in a pot. Add cabbage, cover, and reduce flame to medium. Simmer 4 minutes or so. The cooked cabbage should be bright green and slightly crisp. Remove from water. Mix in chopped parsley and place in a serving bowl. Serve.

Cherry Strudel

1 teaspoon kuzu
¼ cup water
3 cups fresh cherries, washed and pitted
2 tablespoons water
pinch of sea salt
½ cup chopped almonds
pie dough (see page 162)

Place 1 teaspoon of kuzu in ¼ cup water to dilute it, making sure to dissolve all lumps. Place cherries in a pot and add about 2 tablespoons of water and a pinch of sea salt. On a low flame bring to a boil. Simmer 3–5 minutes. Mix diluted kuzu in very well to coat all the cherries. Simmer until kuzu has formed a thick sauce. Remove from flame and mix in chopped almonds. Allow to cool.

Roll out prepared pastry dough as you would if making a pie crust. When cherry mixture has cooled, spoon it onto the rolled out pastry dough. Spread evenly to cover, leaving only the edges of the pastry uncovered. Roll the filled pastry into a log shape or cylinder. Seal the ends of the roll shut by pressing down on the pastry with a wet fork. Poke several holes in the top of the roll with a fork to let steam escape while cooking and to keep the strudel from splitting in half. Oil a baking sheet and place strudel on it. Bake at 375° F for about 30 minutes or until crust is golden brown. Remove and allow strudel to cool. Slice into 1½-to-2-inch rounds. Serve rounds on a platter, with sliced edges facing up.

DAY 7

BREAKFAST MENU

Soft Millet and Sweet Corn

Onion-Shoyu Pickles

Bancha Tea or Grain Coffee
(see page 30)

Soft Millet and Sweet Corn

1 cup millet
1 cup sweet corn, removed from cob
4–5 cups water
pinch of sea salt
green nori flakes

Wash millet. Place millet, sweet corn, and water in a pot and add a pinch of sea salt. Bring to a boil, reduce flame to low, and cover. Simmer 30–35 minutes. Garnish with green nori flakes and serve.

Onion-Shoyu Pickles

2 cups onions, thinly sliced in half-moons
1–2 tablespoons shoyu soy sauce
1–2 tablespoons brown rice vinegar
   (optional)

Slice onions and place in a bowl. Pour shoyu and brown rice vinegar over onions and mix very well to coat all the onions. Let onions sit for about 2 hours or so and then rinse and serve. You may leave these overnight to pickle longer. These pickles will keep about 1 week in a cool place.

LUNCH MENU

❧

Somen with Cool Broth

Boiled Watercress Garnish

Toasted Nori Strips

Bancha Tea
(see page 30)

Somen with Cool Broth

8 ounces (dry weight) whole-wheat
somen noodles
1 strip kombu, 2 inches long, soaked 2–3
minutes in 1 cup water
3 shiitake mushrooms, soaked 7–10 min-
utes in cold water to cover, stems
removed, and sliced
4–5 cups water for broth
3–4 tablespoons shoyu soy sauce

Bring a pot of water to a boil and place the noodles in it. Cook until done. Remove, rinse under cold water, and drain. Place kombu and shiitake in a pot with 4–5 cups of cold water. Bring to a boil. Cover, reduce flame to medium-low, and simmer about 10 minutes. Remove kombu and set it aside for use in other dishes. Season broth with shoyu soy sauce, cover, and reduce flame to low. Simmer 5 minutes. Remove and allow to cool at room temperature or in the refrigerator.

Place the noodles in 4 or 5 serving bowls. Pour cool shoyu broth over each individual serving. Garnish each bowl with Boiled Watercress and Toasted Nori Strips (see page 121).

Boiled Watercress Garnish

2–3 cups water
1 bunch watercress

Place 2–3 cups of water in a pot and bring to a boil. Drop in the watercress, moving it around to cook evenly. Boil for about 45 seconds. Remove, drain, and spread watercress out on a plate to cool. Place a few sprigs of cress as a garnish on each bowl of Somen with Cool Broth.

Toasted Nori Strips

1 sheet nori

Toasted nori goes well with many dishes and is often used as a garnish. To toast nori for general use, turn flame to high and hold a sheet of nori 10–12 inches above the flame so that the inside fold faces downward. Rotate sheet above flame so that it toasts evenly; in a few seconds, it will change from dark to bright green in color. Cut toasted nori into quarters crosswise. Then cut each strip into smaller strips about 2 inches long by ¼ inch wide.

DINNER MENU

Brown Rice Salad

Azuki Beans

Miso Soup with Tofu

Arame with Sweet Corn and Onions

Boiled Turnip Greens with Sesame Seeds

Fresh Cantaloupe Slices

Brown Rice Salad

2 cups brown rice
pinch of sea salt per cup of rice
2½–3 cups of water
1 cup carrots, diced and parboiled
1 cup fresh green peas, parboiled
½ cucumber, quartered and sliced
½ cup celery, diced
2 shiso leaves, rinsed and chopped very fine
2 tablespoons chopped scallions, chives, or parsley

Wash rice and pressure-cook as directed on page 46. When rice is done, remove it from pressure cooker and place in a bowl to cool. Fluff rice to make it lighter and to remove steam.

Place a small amount of water in a saucepan and boil carrots and peas separately until done. Remove and allow to cool.

Mix cucumber, celery, carrots, and peas in with rice. Mix finely chopped shiso leaves in with rice and vegetables, making sure shiso is evenly distributed. Garnish with scallions, chives, or parsley and serve.

Azuki Beans

1 cup azuki beans, washed and soaked for 6–8 hours
water
⅛ teaspoon sea salt
parsley

Place azuki in a pot and add water to cover. Bring to a boil. Reduce flame to medium-low, cover, and simmer for about 2 hours, occasionally adding water to the beans as they need it. After about 2 hours, season the beans with sea salt. Cook until most of the remaining liquid is gone. Place in a serving bowl, garnish with a sprig of fresh parsley, and serve.

Miso Soup with Tofu

⅛ cup wakame, soaked and chopped
3 shiitake mushrooms, soaked, stems
    removed, and sliced
4–5 cups water
1 cup turnips, sliced
1 cake (16 ounces) tofu, cubed
½–1 teaspoon puréed barley miso per cup
    of liquid
sliced scallions
½ teaspoon fresh grated ginger

Place wakame, shiitake, and water in a pot. Bring to a boil. Reduce flame to medium-low, cover, and simmer several minutes. Add turnip slices. Simmer until turnips are soft. Add tofu. Reduce flame to very low and add a small amount of puréed barley miso. Simmer 2–3 minutes. Place in individual serving bowls and garnish each bowl with scallion slices and a little freshly grated ginger.

Arame with Sweet Corn and Onions

2 cups arame
dark sesame oil
1 cup onions, sliced in half-moons
water
shoyu soy sauce
1 cup fresh corn, removed from cob

Wash arame and place in a colander to drain. Do not soak it. Heat a small amount of oil in a skillet. Add onions and sauté 1–2 minutes, stirring to cook evenly. Add arame and just enough water to cover onions. Add a small amount of shoyu, cover, and bring to a boil. Reduce flame to medium-low and simmer about 30 minutes or so. Add sweet corn, and if desired, season with a little more shoyu. Simmer until all liquid is gone. Place in a serving bowl and serve.

Boiled Turnip Greens with Sesame Seeds

water
3 cups turnip greens, sliced
2 tablespoons roasted sesame seeds

Place a small amount of water in a pot and bring to a boil. Add turnip greens, cover, and boil 2–3 minutes. Stir occasionally to cook evenly. Remove and drain greens. Place in a serving dish.

Place roasted sesame seeds in a suribachi and grind slightly. Sprinkle over turnip greens and serve.

Fresh Cantaloupe Slices

1 fresh cantaloupe
sea salt

Slice cantaloupe in half and remove seeds. Then slice cantaloupe halves into crescent shapes and arrange them attractively on a platter. You may sprinkle a pinch of sea salt on each melon slice to make it sweeter and juicier. Cantaloupe is often acid tasting, and the salt helps to counteract this.

FOUR

Autumn Cooking

In the autumn, the colors of nature change from bright green to orange, red, brown, yellow, and gold. The leaves eventually fall to the ground. Food is plentiful, and we have many varieties to choose from. The bright natural colors of fall are reflected in the grains, beans, squashes, and vegetables that are readily available in this season.

Millet and round-shaped vegetables such as onions, squashes, and turnips can be prepared often in the autumn and winter, as well as in other seasons. They have the naturally sweet taste that is used most often in macrobiotic cooking. Rice is harvested in the autumn and, like other foods of this season, can be eaten year round. Contracted leafy greens such as daikon, turnips, carrot tops, kale, and autumn fruits can be used more often in the fall.

In the autumn, we serve richer and heartier dishes than in summer, with an emphasis on bean stews, sautéed or deep-fried vegetables, creamy grain stews, sweet rice and mochi, hot amazake, puréed squash soup, squash pies, and others. Vegetables can be more thoroughly cooked in the fall; methods such as nishime, or waterless cooking, and longer-time sautéing, go well with the season, as do dishes like Kimpira Carrots and Burdock. Your sea vegetable dishes can take on a rich, hearty flavor when prepared with tempeh, dried tofu, soybeans, carrots, parsnips, or onions. Autumn dishes are generally seasoned with a little more salt and oil than are summer dishes, and in autumn we use fewer raw foods, frequently serving lightly boiled salads and a variety of autumn greens instead. Our approach to cutting vegetables also changes in the fall. Larger-sized chunks and rounds can be used more often.

DAY 1

BREAKFAST MENU

❦

Soft Rice with Squash

Turnip-Kombu Pickles

Bancha Tea or Grain Coffee
(see page 30)

Soft Rice with Squash

1 cup rice
1 cup squash or Hokkaido pumpkin,
washed and cubed (leave skin on if
unwaxed and organically grown)
5 cups water
pinch of sea salt per cup of rice
sliced scallions and toasted nori strips

Wash rice and place in a pressure cooker. Add cubed squash, water, and sea salt. Cover pressure cooker and bring to pressure. When pressure is up, place a flame deflector under cooker and reduce flame to medium-low. Cook for 50 minutes. Remove from flame and allow pressure to come down. When pressure is down, remove cover and place rice and squash in individual serving dishes. If you have time, you can simmer this dish on a low flame all night instead of pressure-cooking it. Garnish with a few scallion slices and several strips of toasted nori (see page 121). Serve hot.

Turnip-Kombu Pickles

2 cups turnips
1 strip kombu, 4–5 inches long, soaked in
*   1 cup water for 5–7 minutes*
1 teaspoon sea salt

Wash turnips and quarter them. Next, slice each quarter very thin. If the slices are thick, the turnips will not pickle properly. (In general, short-time pickles should either be sliced very thin or chopped very fine.) Place turnips in a pickle press or bowl. Soak kombu for 5–7 minutes or just until soft enough to slice. Slice kombu very thin and mix it in with turnips. Mix sea salt in well with turnips and kombu. Place top on pickle press and press down. If water from pickles rises above the lid, release some of the pressure. Let pickles sit for at least 1–2 days. They will keep for about 1 week if kept cool.

LUNCH MENU

☙

Rice Balls Rolled in Toasted Sesame Seeds

Vegetable Salad with Vinegar-Ginger-
Shoyu Sauce

Grain Coffee
(see page 30)

Rice Balls Rolled in Toasted Sesame Seeds

4–5 cups cooked brown rice
2 umeboshi plums
1 cup toasted sesame seeds
1 sprig watercress or parsley

Place 1 cup of rice in your hand and form it into a ball. Pack tightly. Poke a hole into the center of the rice ball and insert about ¼ umeboshi plum. Pack the rice ball again to close the hole. You may need to moisten your hands with a little cold water to keep the rice from sticking to them. Be careful not to use too much water as it will detract from the taste and cause the rice ball to fall apart. Roll the formed rice ball in toasted sesame seeds until it is completely coated with seeds. Repeat with remaining rice. Arrange attractively on a platter or tray and serve. This recipe will yield 4 or 5 rice balls. You may garnish the serving plate with a sprig of watercress or parsley. For other rice ball variations, see pages 58 and 71.

Vegetable Salad with Vinegar-Ginger-Shoyu Sauce

2¼–3¼ cups water
1 cup onions, sliced in half-moons
1 cup Chinese cabbage, sliced on a diagonal
  about 1 inch wide
1 cup carrots, thinly sliced on a diagonal
1 tablespoon shoyu soy sauce
½ teaspoon freshly grated ginger
1 tablespoon brown rice vinegar

Place 2–3 cups of water in a pot and bring to a boil. Boil onions for about 50 seconds. Remove onions from pot, making sure to reserve the cooking water. Drain onions and place them in a bowl to cool. Boil cabbage for about 1 minute in the water you used to boil the onions. Remove cabbage from pot, again reserving the cooking water. Drain cabbage and place in bowl with onions. Toss the vegetables to help cool them. Repeat this process with carrots.

Mix ¼ cup water, 1 tablespoon shoyu, ½ teaspoon ginger, and 1 tablespoon vinegar in a small bowl. When serving the vegetable salad, pour about 1 tablespoon of sauce over each portion.

DINNER MENU

Boiled Barley

Soybean Stew

Chinese Cabbage Pickles

Peach Crunch

Boiled Barley

1 cup barley
2–2½ cups water
pinch of sea salt
2 teaspoons chopped parsley

Wash barley and place in a pot with water and sea salt. Cover. Bring to a boil. Reduce flame to medium-low and cook for 50 minutes. Remove cover, and place barley in a wooden bowl. Garnish with parsley and serve.

Soybean Stew

1 piece kombu, 2 x 2 inches, soaked and diced
2 shiitake mushrooms, soaked 7–10
  minutes in cold water to cover,
  stems removed, and diced
¼ cup dried daikon, soaked 5–7 minutes
  in ½ cup water, and sliced
½ cup dried tofu, soaked and cubed
½ cup soybeans, washed and soaked 6–8 hours
2 cups water
¼ cup celery, diced
½ cup onions, diced
¼ cup carrots, diced
2 tablespoons burdock, diced
½ cup sweet corn
grated ginger
sea salt or shoyu soy sauce
sliced scallions for garnish

Soaked dried tofu for 10 minutes. Place kombu, shiitake, dried daikon, dried tofu, and soybeans in a pressure cooker. Add 2 cups water, cover, and bring to pressure. When pressure is up, reduce flame to medium-low, and pressure-cook for about 10 minutes. Remove from flame and allow pressure to come down. When all pressure is out, remove cover and layer celery, onions, carrots, burdock, and sweet corn on top of the beans. Add a little more water if necessary and pressure-cook again for 30 minutes. Then remove from flame and bring pressure down. Remove cover, add a little fresh grated ginger and a little shoyu or sea salt. Simmer 5 minutes more over a medium-low flame. Place in individual serving bowls and garnish with a few sliced scallions. Serve hot.

If you have time and wish to boil these beans instead of pressure cooking them, simmer on a medium-low flame for 3–4 hours, and then add celery, onions, carrots, burdock, and corn. Then boil again for about 1 more hour. Add ginger and seasoning and serve with sliced scallions.

Chinese Cabbage Pickles

1 head Chinese cabbage
¼–⅓ cup sea salt
red pepper

Remove leaves from a head of cabbage and wash individually. Place leaves on a clean dish towel to dry. When water has drained off, cabbage is ready to use. Sprinkle a thin layer of sea salt in the bottom of a ceramic crock or wooden keg. Add a pinch of red pepper. Layer whole cabbage leaves and sea salt with a pinch of red pepper between each layer. Alternate salt, pepper, cabbage, salt, pepper, cabbage, salt, pepper, cabbage, etc., until all the cabbage leaves are used up. The bottom layer and the top layer should always be salt. Use very little pepper, as it makes the cabbage quite hot.

Position the first layer of leaves so that all stems point in the same direction (call this direction north). Position the second layer so that the new leaves cross the first layer at a 90° angle, stems pointing east. The third layer of leaves should be positioned so that their stems are opposite those of the first layer, pointing south, and the stems of the fourth layer should be opposite those of the second layer, pointing west. Continue layering in this manner until all cabbage leaves have been placed in the crock.

Place a wooden disk or plate on top of the last layer of sea salt. Set several heavy, clean rocks or a heavy weight on top of the plate or disk to press the leaves down. Water should rise up to the level of the plate within 10 hours. If this does not happen, you probably have not used enough sea salt. If the water rises above the plate, remove some pressure so that the water level recedes again. Try to keep the water level just below the plate.

Check the pickles every day to make sure that all is going well. They can be rinsed, sliced, and eaten after 3–4 days, or they can be left a few days longer to produce a hotter taste. Store pickles in a cool, dark place. You can always wash some of the salt from pickles or soak them in warm water to remove salt if you have added too much. If, however, you have not used enough salt to begin with, the pickles will mold and spoil. If you find that the pickles are beginning to spoil, you can add more salt, more pressure, or skim off the mold. If the pickles get very moldy, throw them out or use them in a compost heap and start again.

While these pickles are similar to the Chinese Cabbage Pickles listed on page 111, the red pepper adds a subtle difference in flavor that is especially suited for Autumn cooking.

*P*each Crunch

FILLING
10–12 peaches, washed
  and sliced
pinch of sea salt
1 cup water
2 tablespoons kuzu

Place peach slices, sea salt, and water in a saucepan. Bring to a boil. Cover and reduce flame to low. Simmer about 5 minutes or until peaches are soft. Dilute kuzu in 2 tablespoons of water and add to the peaches, stirring constantly to prevent lumping. Simmer 2–3 minutes or until kuzu is translucent and thick. Place peaches in a baking dish.

TOPPING
1 cup rolled oats
¼ cup walnuts
½ cup almonds
¼ cup sunflower seeds, washed
2 tablespoons brown rice syrup
  or barley malt

For topping, lightly roast oats in a dry skillet on a low flame, until golden brown. Stir constantly to prevent burning. Place roasted oats in a mixing bowl. Then lightly roast each variety of nuts and seeds separately in a dry skillet. Chop walnuts and almonds. Add walnuts, almonds, and sunflower seeds to oats. Mix syrup in well with oat-nut mixture. Sprinkle crunch over peaches.

Place peach crunch in a 350° F oven for about 15–20 minutes or until golden brown. Remove from oven and allow to cool slightly. Serve.

DAY 2

BREAKFAST MENU

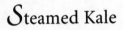

Soft Rice with Umeboshi
(see page 29)

Steamed Kale

Bancha Tea or Grain Coffee
(see page 30)

Steamed Kale

4 cups kale, chopped

Place 2 inches of water in a steamer pot and bring to a boil. Place kale in the steamer, cover, and steam for 2 minutes.

Tempeh Sandwiches

Bancha Tea
(see page 30)

*T*empeh Sandwiches

dark sesame oil
4–5 squares of tempeh, 3 inches x 3 inches
water
shoyu soy sauce
8 or 10 slices whole-wheat bread
  (see page 114)
½ cup sauerkraut (see page 157)
4–5 leaves of lettuce, washed
mustard

Heat a small amount of oil in a skillet. Fry tempeh 1–2 minutes, turn over, and fry other side 1–2 minutes. Add enough water to cover the tempeh halfway. Season with a little shoyu. Cover, reduce flame to medium-low, and simmer about 15–20 minutes. Remove cover and cook until remaining water is gone. Remove tempeh and place on 4 or 5 slices of bread. Place about 1 tablespoon of sauerkraut, a little mustard, and a lettuce leaf on top of each square of tempeh. Add remaining slices of bread to form sandwiches. Slice and place on a serving platter or tray. Serve.

DINNER MENU

❧

Millet with Squash

Yu-Dofu

Miso Soup with Deep-Fried Croutons

Kimpira Carrots and Burdock

Arame with Lotus Root

Amazake Pudding

Millet with Squash

2 cups millet
2 cups butternut squash, washed
    and diced
6 cups water
pinch of sea salt per cup of millet
2 teaspoons chopped parsley

Wash millet and dry-roast in a skillet until golden. Place millet and squash in a pot. Add water and sea salt. Cover and bring to a boil. Reduce the flame to medium-low and simmer 30–35 minutes. Remove from flame. Remove cover, place millet and squash in a wooden bowl, garnish with parsley, and serve. You may wish to prepare a little extra Millet with Squash, because if there is some left over, it can be used for Day 3 Lunch, Millet and Squash Stew (page 142).

Yu-Dofu

1 strip kombu, 2 inches long
4 shiitake mushrooms, sliced
2 cups water
2 cakes (16 ounces each) fresh tofu
2 bunches watercress
finely sliced scallions

Place kombu, shiitake, and 2 cups of water in a saucepan and bring to a boil. Reduce flame to low and simmer several minutes. Remove kombu and set aside for use in soups and other dishes. Let the stock simmer on a low flame while preparing tofu.

Drain tofu and slice it into 1-inch-thick slices. Place drained, sliced tofu in the pot. Slowly bring tofu to a simmer on a medium flame. (If a high flame is used, the tofu will become hard.) When tofu is warm, dip washed watercress into the hot liquid for a few seconds. Serve 2 or 3 slices of tofu and watercress to each person.

Miso Soup with Deep-Fried Croutons

⅛ cup wakame, soaked and sliced
4–5 cups water
2 cups onions, sliced in half-moons
½–1 teaspoon puréed miso per cup
  of liquid
½ cup whole-wheat bread cubes
  (1 slice of bread)
light sesame oil for deep frying
sliced scallions

Soak wakame for 3–5 minutes. Place wakame and onions in water and simmer until they are soft and tender. Reduce flame to very low, add a little puréed miso, and simmer soup for 2–3 minutes.

Slice whole-wheat bread into cubes and deep-fry in hot sesame oil until golden brown. Remove croutons and drain.

Place miso soup in individual serving bowls and garnish with some scallion slices and a few croutons. Serve hot.

Kimpira Carrots and Burdock

1 cup burdock, cut into matchsticks
    or shaved
2 cups carrots, cut into matchsticks
water
shoyu soy sauce
sliced scallions

Cover the bottom of a skillet with a small amount of water. Add burdock. Bring to a boil and boil 1–2 minutes. Add carrots, cover, and cook. Use a high flame to keep the vegetables crisp. Cook until vegetables are just slightly crisp. Season with a little shoyu and cook remaining liquid off. Garnish with a few sliced scallions. Place in a serving dish and serve.

Arame with Lotus Root

dark sesame oil
1 cup fresh lotus root, rounds sliced into
    strips ⅛ inch thick
1 ounce arame, washed and drained
water
shoyu soy sauce

Heat a small amount of dark sesame oil in a skillet. Sauté sliced lotus root 2–3 minutes. Place arame on top of lotus slices. Add enough water to cover lotus root but not arame. Add a small amount of shoyu soy sauce and bring to a boil. Cover and reduce flame to low. Simmer about 45 minutes. Season with a little more shoyu for a mild salt taste. Continue simmering until all liquid is gone. Mix and place in a serving dish. Serve.

*A*mazake Pudding

1 quart amazake drink
6 tablespoons kuzu, diluted with 5–6
  tablespoons water
1 lemon slice for garnish
2 small celery or parsley leaves
  for garnish

Stir amazake and diluted kuzu into a pot. Slowly bring to a boil, stirring constantly to prevent lumping and burning. Simmer several minutes and pour into a serving dish. Smooth out the amazake so that it is evenly distributed in the dish. Garnish with a slice of lemon and a couple of fresh green leaves in the center of the dish. Allow to set. Serve. If enough kuzu is used to thicken the amazake, it will harden and can be sliced into squares to serve. Otherwise, spoon out to serve.

DAY 3

BREAKFAST MENU

ↄ

Miso Soup with Squash Skins

Boiled Tempeh

Bancha Tea or Grain Coffee
(see page 30)

$\mathcal{M}$iso Soup with Squash Skins

4–5 cups water
⅛ cup wakame, soaked and sliced
1 cup onions, sliced in half-moons
1 cup buttercup squash skins, cut into
*   matchsticks (use skins from organi-*
*   cally grown, unwaxed squash)*
2–3 teaspoons puréed barley miso
sliced scallions

Place water in a pot and bring to a boil. Add wakame, onions, and squash skins. Save the fleshy part of the squash for use in Puréed Squash Soup (see page 143). Reduce flame to medium-low and simmer until onions are translucent and soft and squash skins are tender.

Reduce flame to very low and add 2–3 teaspoons of puréed barley miso. Simmer 2–3 minutes more before spooning soup into individual serving bowls. Garnish each bowl with a few scallion slices and serve.

Boiled Tempeh

8 ounces tempeh
water
shoyu soy sauce
ginger
1 cup sliced scallions

Slice tempeh into 1-inch cubes and place in a saucepan. Add water to almost cover. Bring to a boil. Reduce flame to medium-low and simmer about 15 minutes. Add a little shoyu and grated ginger. Simmer 3–4 more minutes. Add sliced scallions and simmer about 1 minute without a cover or until all liquid is gone. Remove and place in a serving bowl. Serve.

L U N C H   M E N U

Millet and Squash Stew

Chinese Cabbage Pickles
(see page 132)

Grain Coffee
(see page 30)

Millet and Squash Stew

5–6 cups water

4–5 cups of cooked millet and squash
(leftovers from Day #2 Dinner work
very well in this dish—see page 136)

1 cup onions, sliced in half-moons
or chunks

1 cup cabbage, sliced into 1-inch chunks

¼ cup chopped scallions or parsley

Place 5–6 cups of water in a pot. Add millet, squash, onions, and cabbage. Bring to a boil. Reduce flame to medium-low, cover, and simmer until vegetables are soft and millet is soft and creamy—about 30–35 minutes. Place in individual serving bowls and garnish with chopped scallions or parsley. Serve hot.

DINNER MENU

Brown Rice with Wild Rice

Puréed Squash Soup

Chinese-Style Sautéed Vegetables

Kombu Carrot Rolls

Kidney Beans with Miso

Brown Rice with Wild Rice

1 cup brown rice
1 cup wild rice
2½–3 cups water
pinch of sea salt per cup of grain
chopped parsley and scallions

Wash brown and wild rice, place in a pressure cooker, and add water. Place on a low flame for 15–20 minutes. Add sea salt, cover, and turn flame to high. Bring to pressure and place a flame deflector under the cooker. Reduce flame to medium-low and pressure-cook for 50 minutes. Remove from flame and bring pressure down. When all pressure is out, remove cover. Let rice sit for about 4–5 minutes and then transfer it to a serving bowl. Garnish with chopped parsley or scallions and serve. You may wish to prepare a little extra Brown Rice with Wild Rice, because if there is some left over, it can be used for Day 4 Lunch, Fried Wild Rice with Tofu and Vegetables (page 147).

Puréed Squash Soup

4 cups buttercup squash or Hokkaido
    pumpkin, without skin or seeds,
    cubed
4–5 cups water
1 cup diced onions
sliced scallions

Place squash cubes in a pot with water. Bring to a boil. Reduce flame to medium-low and cover. Simmer until soft, about 10–15 minutes. Purée squash in a hand food mill and place it back into cooking pot. Add diced onions and bring to a boil. Reduce flame to medium-low and cover. Simmer about 15 minutes. Place in individual serving bowls and garnish each with a few scallion slices. Serve hot.

Chinese-Style Sautéed Vegetables

dark sesame oil
2 cups cabbage, finely sliced
1 cup celery, sliced on a diagonal
pinch of sea salt

Brush a small amount of dark sesame oil in a skillet and heat up. Add cabbage. Sauté 1–2 minutes on a high flame, stirring constantly to prevent burning and to sauté evenly. Add celery and sauté 1–2 minutes. Keep flame high to keep vegetables crisp. Mix in a pinch of sea salt. Continue to sauté for a short time; the vegetables should remain crisp. Remove and place in a serving bowl. Serve.

Kombu Carrot Rolls

2 strips kombu, 12 inches long by
   3 inches wide
2½–3 cups water
4 medium carrots (about 6 inches long)
8 strips kampyo (gourd strips), 6 inches
   long, soaked about 5 minutes
shoyu soy sauce

Soak kombu in about 2½–3 cups water for about 5–7 minutes. Remove kombu and save soaking water. Slice each strip of kombu into 6-inch lengths.

Place a 6-inch length of kombu on a cutting board. Place 1 carrot on the strip and roll it up as tightly as possible. Tie kombu roll in three places, evenly spaced apart. If you do not have kampyo for tying the kombu rolls, simply soak an additional strip of kombu (about 3 inches by 6 inches) for several minutes and slice it into 8 thin strips, about 6 inches long by ¼ inch wide, for tying.

Roll and tie kombu and carrots until all ingredients are used up. Place water from soaking kombu in a pot. Add kombu rolls and bring to a boil. Cover and reduce flame to medium-low. Simmer about 45 minutes to 1 hour. Add a little shoyu and simmer several minutes longer or until kombu and carrots are very tender.

If you wish to save time by pressure-cooking these vegetables, place soaking water and kombu rolls in a pressure cooker. Add a little shoyu and bring to pressure. Reduce flame to medium-low and pressure-cook for about 20–25 minutes.

Remove cooked kombu rolls and slice each 6-inch-long roll into three 2-inch-long sections. (When slicing, make sure that each section is secured with kampyo.) Arrange sections on a platter and serve.

For variation you can halve or quarter the carrots and halve or quarter some burdock and roll a piece of each inside each strip of kombu.

Kidney Beans with Miso

1 cup kidney beans, washed, and soaked
  for 6–8 hours
water
1–1½ teaspoons puréed barley miso

Place beans in a pot. Add just enough water to cover beans. Bring to a boil. Reduce flame to medium-low and cover. Simmer for about 2 hours. Add water occasionally while cooking, only as needed to just cover beans as they expand and absorb water. After 2 hours or so, place puréed miso on top of beans. Do not mix, because the natural cooking action of the beans will draw the miso down. Continue cooking until beans are soft and creamy. Place in a serving bowl and serve.

Kidney beans are best when cooked several hours over a low flame, but if you have a limited amount of time you may pressure-cook them for 50 minutes instead. Then add puréed miso and simmer about 20–30 minutes longer over low flame.

DAY 4

BREAKFAST MENU

❦

Miso Soup with Wakame and Daikon

Broiled Tofu
(see page 91)

Bancha Tea or Grain Coffee
(see page 30)

Miso Soup with Wakame and Daikon

4–5 cups water
⅛ cup wakame, washed and soaked 2–3
*   minutes, and sliced*
1 cup daikon, cut in thin half-moons
*   or rectangles*
1½–2 tablespoons puréed miso
sliced scallions

Place water in a pot and bring to a boil. Add wakame and daikon. Cover, reduce flame to low, and simmer for about 5 minutes, until the daikon is soft. Reduce flame to very low and add puréed miso. Mix in miso and simmer 1–2 minutes or so. Place soup in individual serving bowls. Garnish with scallion slices and serve hot.

ↄ

Fried Wild Rice with Tofu and Vegetables

Pickled Daikon or Turnip Greens
(see page 44)

Bancha Tea
(see page 30)

*F*ried Wild Rice with Tofu and Vegetables

dark sesame oil
½ cup onion, diced
½ cup celery, diced
1 cup cabbage, cut into 1-inch chunks
4–5 cups cooked wild rice (Leftovers from
   Day #3 Dinner work very well in this
   dish—see page 143)
1 cup fresh tofu
shoyu soy sauce
1 tablespoon chopped parsley

Heat a small amount of dark sesame oil in a skillet. Add onions and sauté 1–2 minutes. Add celery, cabbage, and wild rice. Crumble tofu and place it on top. Cover skillet, reduce flame to very low, and simmer until vegetables are tender and tofu is light and fluffy. Add a small amount of shoyu soy sauce. Cook 2–3 more minutes. Mix. Place in a serving dish and garnish with chopped parsley.

*A*zuki Beans and Squash

1 cup azuki beans, washed and soaked
    6–8 hours
1 cup organically grown, unwaxed but-
    tercup squash or Hokkaido pumpkin,
    washed, seeds removed, and cubed
    (leave skin on)
¼ teaspoon sea salt
water

Place beans in a pot. Place squash on top of beans. Add just enough water to cover squash but not beans. Place on a low flame and slowly bring to a boil. Cook for about 2 hours. Add water occasionally as needed because the beans expand and water evaporates. When beans have cooked for about 2 hours, add sea salt and continue cooking until most of the liquid is gone. Place in a serving bowl and serve.

Cauliflower Clear Soup

2 cups cauliflower florets
4–5 cups water
½ teaspoon sea salt
5–6 sprigs of fresh parsley, minced
5 lemon slices

Place cauliflower, water, and sea salt in a pot, cover, and bring to a boil. Simmer 10–15 minutes. Mash the cauliflower with a potato masher. Ladle into bowls and garnish with parsley and a slice of lemon in each bowl.

Steamed or Boiled Kale

4 cups kale, sliced
water

Steam or boil kale in a small amount of water. It should be bright green when done. You can either slice kale before cooking or use 5–6 whole leaves and slice them after they are cooked.

Baked Apples with Kuzu-Raisin Sauce

1 cup apple juice
¼ cup raisins
pinch of sea salt
1 tablespoon kuzu
1 tablespoon water
5–6 baking apples

Place apple juice, raisins, and sea salt in a saucepan and bring to a boil. Reduce flame to low and simmer, covered, for about 5 minutes. Dilute kuzu in 1 tablespoon of water and add to apple juice and raisins. Stir constantly to prevent lumping. Set aside.

Wash apples (do not peel them) and bake in a baking dish with a little water at 375° F for about 15–20 minutes. To serve, place 1 apple in each individual serving bowl and spoon the kuzu-raisin sauce on top. Serve hot.

DAY 5

BREAKFAST MENU

❦

Soft Millet with Corn and Onions

Onion-Shoyu Pickles
(see page 119)

Bancha Tea or Grain Coffee
(see page 30)

Soft Millet with Corn and Onions

1 cup millet
½ cup onions, diced
½ cup fresh sweet corn, removed from cob
4–5 cups water

pinch of sea salt per cup of grain
green nori flakes or scallion slices

Wash millet and place in a pot with onions and corn. Add water and a pinch of sea salt. Bring to a boil. Reduce flame to medium-low, cover, and simmer for 30–35 minutes. Place in individual serving bowls and garnish each bowl with green nori flakes or scallion slices.

LUNCH MENU

Pan-Fried Rice Croquettes

Shoyu-Ginger Sauce

Boiled Kale

Grain Coffee
(see page 30)

$\mathcal{P}$an-Fried Rice Croquettes

4–5 cups cooked rice
1 cup onions, diced
½ cup carrots, diced
½ cup celery, diced
1 tablespoon chopped parsley
½ cup water (approximately)
dark sesame oil

Place rice, onions, carrots, celery, and parsley in a bowl. Add enough water to hold rice and vegetables together. If rice is very moist to begin with, you may omit water and add a little flour. Mix very well. Take a handful of rice mixture and press it together firmly, forming croquettes. Repeat until all rice is used up. Set croquettes aside.

Heat a little oil in a skillet, cover, and reduce flame to medium-low. Cook until croquettes are golden brown. Turn over and fry other side until golden brown. Remove and place on a serving plate. Serve with Shoyu-Ginger Sauce (below).

Shoyu-Ginger Sauce

½ *cup water*
¼ *cup shoyu*
½ *teaspoon fresh grated ginger*

Mix all ingredients. Spoon sauce over Pan-Fried Rice Croquettes (above), or other vegetable or grain dishes.

Boiled Kale

4 *cups kale, washed and sliced*
on a diagonal
water

Place about 1 inch of water in the bottom of a pot and bring it to a boil. Add kale and cover. Reduce flame to medium-low and simmer 3–4 minutes or until done. Boiled kale is best when it is bright green and slightly crisp. Remove, drain, and place in a serving bowl. Serve.

❧

Sweet Brown Rice and Azuki Beans

Deep-Fried Tofu with Kuzu Sauce

Daikon Clear Soup

Celery, Carrot, Apple, and Dulse Salad

Steamed Kale
(see page 109)

Sweet Brown Rice and Azuki Beans

1 cup azuki beans
3¾–4½ cups of water (approximately)
2 cups sweet brown rice
pinch of sea salt per cup of grain
    and beans
parsley or watercress

Wash azuki beans and place them in a saucepan. Add water to cover beans and bring to a boil. Reduce flame to medium-low and simmer about 15–20 minutes. Remove beans from flame, reserving cooking water, and allow to cool. Use this as part of the water measurement stated above. Instead of boiling, you may soak beans 6–8 hours with water to cover before adding them to rice. Use soaking water as part of the water measurement for rice.

Wash sweet rice after azuki beans and cooking water have cooled sufficiently (it is too much of a sudden shock to add hot water to the rice). Place rice in a pressure cooker. Add beans, bean cooking water, and any additional water needed. Place cooker on low flame for 15–20 minutes. Add sea salt and cover. Turn flame to high and bring up to pressure. Place a flame deflector under the cooker and reduce flame to medium-low. Pressure-cook for 50 minutes. Then remove cooker from flame and bring pressure down. Remove cover and let rice sit for about 4–5 minutes. To serve, spoon rice into a wooden bowl and garnish with a sprig of parsley or watercress.

Deep-Fried Tofu with Kuzu Sauce

1 piece kombu, 2 inches long, soaked
3 cups water
shoyu soy sauce
2 cakes (16 ounces each) fresh tofu
1 cup onions, diced
4 tablespoons kuzu
½ cup sliced scallions
light sesame oil

Place kombu in a pot with 3 cups of water, and bring to a boil. Cover and reduce flame to medium-low. Simmer about 10 minutes. Remove kombu and set it aside for future use. Season water with a little shoyu.

Drain tofu and slice into 1-inch-thick slices. Deep-fry each slice until golden brown. Drain on paper towels.

Place deep-fried tofu and diced onions in the shoyu-seasoned water and simmer for 15–20 minutes. After onions are soft, remove tofu and place it in a serving dish. Reserve the shoyu-seasoned broth with the onions in it. Dilute kuzu in 3 to 4 tablespoons cold water and add it to the shoyu-seasoned hot broth to make a kuzu sauce. Add the sliced scallions to the hot kuzu sauce and pour it over the deep-fried tofu. Serve.

Daikon Clear Soup

4 shiitake mushrooms, soaked and sliced
4–5 cups water
2 cups daikon, sliced
sea salt
¼ cup sliced scallions
1 sheet nori, toasted and cut into strips

Soak shiitake for 10–15 minutes and slice. Place shiitake in water in a pot, cover, and bring to a boil. Reduce flame to medium-low and simmer for 10 minutes. Add daikon and sea salt. Cover, and simmer for 5–7 minutes, or until soft. Pour soup into individual serving bowls and garnish each bowl with scallions and several strips of toasted nori. Serve.

Celery, Carrot, Apple, and Dulse Salad

water
2 cups carrots, halved lengthwise and
    sliced on a diagonal
1 cup celery, sliced on a diagonal
¼ cup dulse, washed, soaked 2–3 minutes,
    and sliced
2 cups sliced apples

Place a little water in a pot and bring to a boil. Reduce flame to medium-low, add carrots, and cook 1½–2 minutes, or until soft. Remove carrots and place in a bowl, reserving the cooking water. Add celery to cooking water and simmer 1½–2 minutes. Celery should remain slightly crisp. Remove celery from flame, drain, and mix in with carrots. Mix in dulse and apples. Place in a serving bowl and serve.

DAY 6

BREAKFAST MENU

ↄ

Soft Bulgur with Scallions

Sauerkraut

Bancha Tea or Grain Coffee
(see page 30)

Soft Bulgar with Scallions

4–5 cups water
1 cup bulgur
pinch of sea salt per cup of bulgur
sliced scallions

Bring 4–5 cups of water to a boil. Add bulgur and sea salt. Bring to a boil, cover, and reduce flame to medium-low. Simmer for 30 minutes or until very soft and creamy. When done place in individual serving bowls and garnish each bowl with a few scallion slices. Serve.

Sauerkraut

5 pounds cabbage
⅓ cup sea salt

Wash and finely shred cabbage. Place it in a wooden keg or ceramic crock. Mix sea salt in very well. Place several clean rocks or a heavy weight on top of a plate or wooden disk to press the cabbage. Cover keg or crock with a piece of clean cheesecloth or cotton linen to keep dust out. Within 10 hours the water level in the keg should be up to or above the plate. If the level is above the plate, remove some of the weight to make the water recede. Keep sauerkraut in a dark cool place for about 1½–2 weeks. Check it every day to make sure all is going well. If mold begins to form on top, make sure to remove and discard it as soon as you notice it. If mold is not removed, it will cause the entire batch of sauerkraut to spoil.

Before placing sauerkraut in a serving dish, rinse it with cold water.

Prepared organic sauerkraut can be purchased at most natural-food stores.

LUNCH MENU

Boiled Seitan

Steamed Cabbage

Bancha Tea
(see page 30)

Boiled Seitan

3½ pounds of whole-wheat flour
18–20 cups spring water
1 piece kombu, 2 inches long, soaked 5–7
*   minutes in 2 cups water*
3–5 tablespoons shoyu soy sauce

Place flour in large bowl and add 8–9 cups of warm water for a consistency like thick oatmeal or cookie batter. Knead for 3–5 minutes until flour is mixed thoroughly with water. Cover with 4–5 cups of warm water and allow to sit a minimum of 5–10 minutes. Knead again in soaking water for 1 minute. Pour off cloudy water into a jar. This cloudy water is the seitan starch water called for in recipes in this book.

Place remaining gluten into a large strainer and put strainer in a large bowl or pot. Pour cold water over gluten and knead in the strainer. Repeat until bran and starch are completely separated. Keep the starch. Alternate between cold and hot water when rinsing and kneading gluten.

Gluten should form a sticky mass. Separate it into 5 or 6 pieces and form balls. Drop balls into 6 cups boiling water and boil for 5 minutes, or until balls rise to surface. Place kombu and shoyu in the boiling water with the gluten balls and cook for 35–45 minutes. The liquid in the pot is the seitan-shoyu water called for in recipes in this book.

Seitan balls can be sliced or cubed for use in various recipes.

Seitan can be stored in shoyu cooking water in a sealed glass jar and kept in the refrigerator for 4 to 5 days. The stronger the concentration of tamari the longer it stores. Seitan stored in full-strength shoyu will keep several weeks but must be soaked in water for about 30 minutes before use, to remove excess salt.

Steamed Cabbage

water
4 cups cabbage, cut in chunks
1 tablespoon roasted sesame seeds

Place about 1 inch of water in a pot and bring to a boil. Add cabbage and cook 3–4 minutes; it should remain slightly crisp. Remove, drain, and place in a serving bowl. Serve garnished with sesame seeds.

DINNER MENU

❧

Millet and Vegetables

Goma Wakame Condiment

Creamy Barley Soup
(see page 46)

Nishime Vegetables with Tofu

Sautéed Bok Choy

Squash Pie

Millet and Vegetables

1 tablespoon sesame oil
½ cup onions, diced
½ cup carrots, diced
2 cups millet, washed
6 cups water
pinch of sea salt per cup of millet

Heat oil in a heavy pot. Sauté onions and carrots 2–3 minutes. Sauté millet 5 minutes, add water and sea salt; cover, and bring to a boil. Reduce flame to medium-low. Cook for 30–35 minutes. Remove from flame and place millet in a wooden serving bowl. Garnish with a sprig of parsley, chopped scallions, roasted sunflower seeds, toasted nori strips, carrot flowers or carrot strips, or another macrobiotic garnish.

Goma Wakame Condiment

1 ounce dry wakame
¼–½ cup sesame seeds, roasted

Place dry wakame in a 350° F oven for about 15–20 minutes or until crisp and dark. Be careful not to burn wakame as a burned flavor will detract from the condiment. Place wakame in a suribachi and grind to a fine powder. Add roasted sesame seeds and grind until seeds are about half crushed. (Grind wakame before grinding the seeds; otherwise the seeds will be ground too fine.) Store the condiment in a sealed jar. Make sure that it cools sufficiently before placing it in a jar, as water will condense in the jar if it is too warm.

Other sea vegetables such as kombu, dulse, and kelp can be used instead of wakame to create different condiments. The proportion of seeds should be about 60 percent and sea vegetables about 40 percent. To use, sprinkle on rice, other grains, or vegetables.

Nishime Vegetables with Tofu

1 square-inch kombu
1 cup deep-fried tofu, cubed
1 cup daikon, halved or cut into thick
  rounds
1 cup fresh lotus root, sliced into rounds
water
shoyu soy sauce

Place kombu in the bottom of a pot. On top of kombu, add deep-fried tofu cubes, daikon, and lotus root. These vegetables should be arranged so that each has its own section of the pot. Daikon on one side, lotus on another, and tofu on another. Add water to cover the vegetables halfway. Bring to a boil. Cover, reduce flame to medium-low, and simmer about 30–35 minutes. Add a little shoyu and simmer about 15 minutes longer or until almost all liquid is gone. Just before removing vegetables, mix them gently. This will coat the vegetables with the juice from cooking. Place in a serving bowl and serve.

Sautéed Bok Choy

dark sesame oil
3 cups bok choy, sliced
sea salt

Heat a small amount of dark sesame oil in a skillet. Add bok choy and a pinch of sea salt. Sauté several minutes. The vegetables should be slightly crisp when done. Place in a serving bowl and serve.

Squash Pie

1 medium buttercup squash
1 cup water
pinch of sea salt
¼–½ cup barley malt
1 tablespoon kuzu
1 cup chopped walnuts

Wash squash and remove skin and seeds. Cut into chunks and place in a pot with 1 cup of water and a pinch of sea salt. Bring to a boil. Reduce flame to medium-low and cover. Simmer until squash is soft. Then purée squash in a hand food mill. Place puréed squash in a pot and add barley malt. Simmer about 5 minutes. Dilute kuzu in 1 tablespoon of water and add it to the puréed squash, stirring constantly to prevent lumping. Simmer 2–3 minutes. Remove from flame and allow to cool.

Pie Dough
2 cups whole-wheat pastry flour
⅛ teaspoon sea salt
⅛ cup corn or sesame oil
⅜–½ cup cold water
chopped walnuts

Mix flour and sea salt together. Add oil to the flour and mix it in well by sifting it with your hands. Add water and form flour into a ball of dough. Knead for about 2–3 minutes. Let it sit for about 5–10 minutes before rolling it out.

Roll out pastry dough and place pastry in a pie plate. With a fork, seal the edges of the crust and poke several small holes in the bottom to let air escape and to keep the crust from buckling. Bake crust at 350° F for about 10 minutes. Remove empty pie shell and pour in squash filling. Smooth out the top of the filling and sprinkle chopped walnuts on top. Bake again for about 30–35 minutes or until pie crust is golden brown.

DAY 7

BREAKFAST MENU

☙

Miso Soup with Wakame and Cauliflower

Toasted Sourdough Bread

Carrot Butter

Bancha Tea or Grain Coffee
(see page 30)

Miso Soup with Wakame and Cauliflower

4–5 cups water
⅛ cup wakame, washed, soaked 2–3
   minutes, and sliced
2 cups cauliflower florets
½–1 teaspoon puréed barley miso
   per cup of liquid
chopped parsley

Place water in a pot and bring to a boil. Add wakame and cauliflower. Cover and reduce flame to medium-low. Simmer until cauliflower is done. Reduce flame to very low and add puréed miso. Simmer 2–3 minutes. Place in individual serving bowls and garnish each bowl with chopped parsley.

Toasted Sourdough Bread

A delicious sourdough starter for bread can be made by combining 1 cup of whole-wheat flour and enough water to make a thick batter. Cover with a damp cloth and allow to ferment for 3–4 days in a warm place. After starter has soured, add 1–1½ cups of starter to bread dough (see page 114), knead, and proceed as for whole-wheat bread. For rye bread, use 3 cups rye flour to 5 cups whole-wheat flour.

Toasted sourdough bread goes well with carrot butter (below) and other spreads, apple butter, or unsweetened jelly. Serve 1 or 2 slices of toasted sourdough bread to each person.

Carrot Butter

dark sesame oil
10 cups carrots, diced
pinch of sea salt
water

Lightly oil a skillet and heat. Sauté carrots on a medium-low flame for several minutes. Transfer sautéed carrots to a pot and add sea salt and just enough water to cover carrots. Bring to a boil. Cover and reduce flame to low. Simmer several hours, until carrots become dark and sweet. If you need more water, occasionally add small quantities while the carrots cook, but avoid using too much water. When carrot butter is done, spread it on your favorite bread, toast, or rice cakes. To store, allow to cool, place in a glass jar, and seal tightly. Carrot butter will keep 1 week at room temperature, 1 month if refrigerated.

Steamed Mochi and Chinese Cabbage

Sautéed Vegetables

Grain Coffee

(see page 30)

Steamed Mochi and Chinese Cabbage

water
4 whole Chinese cabbage leaves
8 pieces of brown rice mochi, 2 inches by
   3 inches

Place half of water in a steamer pot. Bring to a boil. Place cabbage leaves in the steamer. Place 2 pieces of mochi on top of each leaf. Steam 3–4 minutes until mochi melts. Serve.

Sautéed Vegetables

dark sesame oil
½ cup carrots, sliced thinly on a diagonal
1½ cups kale, washed and sliced on a
   diagonal
pinch of sea salt

Heat a small amount of oil in a skillet. Sauté carrots 1–2 minutes. Add kale and sauté 3–4 minutes. Season with a pinch of sea salt and continue to sauté about another minute, so that vegetables remain slightly crisp and kale is bright green. Place in a serving dish and serve.

DINNER MENU

Brown Rice

Seitan Squash Stew

Arame with Lotus Seeds

Steamed Collard Greens

*B*rown Rice

2 cups brown rice, washed
2½–3 cups water
pinch of sea salt per cup of grain

Place rice and water in a pressure cooker. Place on a low flame for 15–20 minutes. Add sea salt. Cover and bring up to pressure. Place a flame deflector under cooker and reduce flame to medium-low. Cook for 50 minutes. Then release pressure and let rice sit for about 4–5 minutes. Transfer cooked rice to a wooden bowl, garnish, and serve.

Seitan Squash Stew

½ cup celery, sliced in thick diagonals
1 cup onions, sliced in quarters or eighths
1 cup squash (buttercup, butternut, or
other winter squash), cubed
1 cup carrots, cut into chunks
2 cups cooked seitan, cut into chunks
3–4 cups seitan-shoyu cooking water
(see Seitan, page 158)
1½ cups seitan-starch water (see Seitan,
page 158)
grated ginger and scallion slices

Place celery, onions, squash, carrots, and seitan in a pot. Pour in seitan-shoyu cooking water. Bring to a boil. Reduce flame to medium-low, cover, and simmer until vegetables are very soft and tender. Reduce flame to low and add seitan-starch water. Stir constantly while you add this water. Simmer stew another 20 minutes or so. The seitan-starch water will cause the stew to become very thick. Place in individual serving bowls and garnish each bowl with a little grated ginger and a few scallion slices. Serve hot.

Arame with Lotus Seeds

1 ounce (about 1½–2 cups) arame
dark sesame oil
1 cup lotus seeds, soaked 4–5 hours
1 cup carrots, matchsticks
water
shoyu

Wash arame and drain, but do not soak it as it may lose flavor and nutrients. Heat a small amount of dark sesame oil in a skillet. Add arame and sauté 2–3 minutes. Add lotus seeds, carrots, and water to half cover arame and seeds. Add a small amount of shoyu and bring to a boil. Cover and reduce flame to medium-low. Simmer about 40–45 minutes. Add a little more shoyu and continue to cook until almost all liquid is gone and lotus seeds are very soft (10–15 minutes). Mix. Place in a serving dish and serve.

Steamed Collard Greens

water
3 cups collard greens, sliced

Place a small amount of water in a pot and bring to a boil. Set collard greens in a steamer in the pot and steam several minutes until done. They should be bright green and slightly crisp. Remove and place in a serving dish.

FIVE

Winter Cooking

We need warm, strong food during the cold winter months. Our food provides us with the warmth and strength that we need to endure the extreme cold weather.

In winter, meals may be more strongly seasoned than at any other time of year. Nevertheless, be careful not to use too much sea salt, shoyu, or miso in your winter cooking. The moderate use of seasoning is preferable at all times of year.

A little more oil is needed for winter cooking than for autumn. Dishes such as deep-fried grains, tempura, sautéed vegetables, and kimpira can be included more often, and a little more oil and shoyu can be used in preparing sea vegetables. Fried rice and noodles are also good, together with stronger miso soups and grain, bean, seitan, and vegetable stews. Sweet brown rice and mochi can be served more frequently in the winter than in other seasons. They contain more protein and fat than regular brown rice and help to produce a warming effect.

Longer cooking methods are generally appropriate in the winter, including nishime-style vegetables, baked grain, bean, and vegetable dishes, and well-sautéed vegetable dishes.

However, do not let your cooking become one-sided. Quick, light cooking methods and fresh greens can be used for variety in any season, including winter.

As winter progresses and spring approaches, we begin to lighten our cooking to harmonize with the energy of the coming season. In this way we harmonize our blood quality and overall condition with the natural cycle of change. This is the art of macrobiotic cooking.

DAY 1

Miso Soup with Wakame and Daikon
(see page 33)

*Boiled Tofu with Tamari, Ginger,
and Scallions*

Bancha Tea or Grain Coffee
(see page 30)

*B*oiled Tofu with Tamari, Ginger, and Scallions

2 cakes (16 ounces each) tofu, quartered
water
shoyu soy sauce
grated ginger
¼ cup sliced scallions

Place a small amount of cold water in a saucepan. Place on a medium-low flame. Add tofu. Heat the water slowly to keep the tofu soft. If you use a high flame, the tofu will harden. When tofu is warmed, place 1–2 pieces on each person's plate. Garnish each piece of tofu with a couple of drops of shoyu, a pinch of ginger, and a few scallion slices. Serve.

Boiled Fu with Tofu, Broccoli, and Carrots

Bancha Tea
(see page 30)

Boiled Fu with Tofu, Broccoli, and Carrots

4-ounce package fu,
   soaked and sliced
½ cup carrots, sliced on
   a diagonal
water
2 cups broccoli florets
4-ounces fresh tofu, cubed
shoyu soy sauce

Place fu and carrots in a pot. Add enough water to about half cover. Bring to a boil. Cover, reduce flame to medium-low, and simmer about 2–3 minutes. Add broccoli and simmer about 2–3 minutes more. Add tofu and shoyu soy sauce to taste. Simmer 1–2 minutes longer. Remove and place in a serving dish. Serve hot.

*B*rown Rice and Azuki Beans

2 cups brown rice
1 cup azuki beans, washed, parboiled,
   and cooled
3¾–4½ cups water, including water
   from cooking beans
pinch of sea salt per cup of rice

Wash rice and place in pressure cooker. Add cool azuki beans and water from cooking beans. Place pressure cooker on low flame for 15–20 minutes. Add sea salt and place cover on cooker. Turn flame to high and bring up to pressure. Place a flame deflector under cooker, reduce flame to medium-low, and cook 50 minutes. Remove from flame and bring down pressure. Remove cover and let rice sit for 4–5 minutes before serving in a wooden bowl. You may wish to prepare a little extra Brown Rice and Azuki Beans, because if there is some left over, it can be used for Day 2 Lunch, Rice and Azuki Bean Stew (page 177).

Seitan Barley Stew

1 shiitake mushroom, soaked 7–10 minutes
  in cold water to cover, and diced
¼ cup celery, diced
1 cup onions, diced
1 tablespoon scallion root and additional
  scallion slices for garnish
½ cup dried daikon, soaked 5–7 minutes
  in ½ cup water and diced in 1-inch
  lengths
½ cup cabbage, sliced
1 cup carrots, diced
1 cup boiled seitan (see page 158), cubed
¼ cup burdock, diced or quartered
½ cup barley, soaked 6–8 hours
8 cups water, including soaking water
  from barley

Place shiitake, celery, onions, scallion root, dried daikon, cabbage, carrots, seitan, and burdock in layers in a pot. Use the order of layering or adding vegetables listed above for best results. Place soaked barley on top of the burdock layer. Add water to just cover barley (and vegetables). Bring to a boil. Cover and reduce flame to medium-low. Simmer until barley and vegetables are very soft. If you have time, continue to simmer on a low flame until barley becomes very soft and creamy. It becomes very delicious then. If necessary, after the barley is soft, add shoyu or sea salt to suit your taste, and cook 5–10 more minutes. Place stew in individual serving bowls and garnish each bowl with a few scallion slices. Serve hot.

Arame with Dried Tofu and Carrots

water
1 ounce arame (about 1½–2 cups)
1 cup dried tofu
1 cup carrots, cut in matchsticks
dark sesame oil
shoyu soy sauce

Place 2 cups of water on to boil. While waiting, wash arame and drain it in a colander, but do not soak. Next place dried tofu in a bowl and pour the boiling water over it. Soak dried tofu until soft (2–3 minutes). Then rinse under cold water and squeeze out liquid. Cube tofu and set it aside. Heat a small amount of dark sesame oil in a skillet, add arame and carrots, and sauté 1–2 minutes. Add tofu, water to half-cover arame and carrots, and a small amount of shoyu. Bring to a boil. Cover and reduce flame to low. Simmer 40–45 minutes. Season with a little more shoyu and simmer another 10–15 minutes. Almost all the liquid should be cooked away. Mix all ingredients. Place in a serving bowl and serve.

Boiled Collard Greens

water
3 cups chopped collard greens
*   and sliced stems*

Place about ½ inch of water in a pot and bring to a boil. Add collards, cover, and boil about 2–3 minutes. The collards should be bright green and slightly crisp when done. Place in a serving bowl and serve.

DAY 2

BREAKFAST MENU

ↄ

Miso Soft Rice
(see page 43)

Pickled Mustard Greens

Bancha Tea or Grain Coffee
(see page 30)

*P*ickled Mustard Greens

10 whole mustard green leaves,
    washed
sea salt

Place 3 leaves in a pickle press. Sprinkle a pinch of sea salt over them. Place another layer of 3–4 leaves and another pinch of sea salt in the press. Add the remaining leaves and sprinkle another pinch of sea salt on top. Apply pressure by screwing down the press. Leave pickles for 1 to 2 days. If they are too salty, rinse them under cold water before slicing; slice and serve.

Rice and Azuki Bean Stew

Sautéed Chinese Cabbage

Grain Coffee
(see page 30)

Rice and Azuki Bean Stew

4–5 cups cooked Brown Rice and
Azuki Beans (page 173)
5–6 cups water
1 cup daikon, sliced into thin rectangular
shapes
1 cup kale, washed and sliced on
a diagonal
sea salt

Place Brown Rice and Azuki Beans in a pot and add water and daikon. Bring to a boil. Cover, reduce flame to medium-low, and simmer about 35–40 minutes. Add kale and sea salt to taste. Simmer for 2–3 minutes. It is best if the kale is bright green. Serve.

Sautéed Chinese Cabbage

dark sesame oil
4–5 cups Chinese cabbage,
 sliced on a diagonal
sea salt

Heat a small amount of oil in a skillet. Add cabbage and a pinch of sea salt. Sauté 3–4 minutes, stirring constantly to cook evenly. Remove and place in a serving dish. Serve.

DINNER MENU

Gomoku

Tempeh and Onions with Kuzu-Ginger Sauce

Boiled Daikon with Black Sesame Seeds

Boiled Watercress
(see page 65)

Gomoku

2 cups brown rice
½ cup lotus root, diced
½ cup dried tofu, soaked, rinsed, and diced

1 teaspoon scallion root, minced
½ cup dried daikon, soaked and sliced
1 cup carrots, diced
½ cup burdock, diced
2½ cups of water
pinch of sea salt

Wash rice and place in a pressure cooker. Mix in all ingredients very well, add sea salt and 2½ cups of water. Place cover on the pressure cooker. Turn flame to high and bring to pressure. Place a flame deflector under cooker and reduce flame to medium-low. Cook for 50 minutes. After this time, remove from flame and bring pressure down. Remove cover when all pressure is out. Let rice sit for 4–5 minutes to loosen it from the bottom of the pot. Remove and serve in a wooden bowl.

Tempeh and Onions with Kuzu-Ginger Sauce

5–6 whole onions
8 ounces tempeh, cut into
    2-inch-by-1-inch slices
shoyu soy sauce
4–5 cups water (approximately)
4–5 tablespoons kuzu
½ teaspoon fresh grated ginger
chopped parsley

Peel onions and slice an "X" in the top of each one. Place onions and tempeh slices in a heavy pot. Add water to half cover onions. Bring to a boil. Cover and reduce flame to low. Simmer until onions are soft. Add ¼–½ teaspoon shoyu and cook 20 minutes.

Place onions and tempeh in a serving dish and measure the cooking liquid that remains in the pot. If liquid has evaporated and there is less than 4–5 cups, add plain water to equal that amount. Dilute kuzu in ¼ cup of water and add it to the water in the pot. Stir until thick and clear. Season with 2–3 tablespoons shoyu, if desired, and add a little grated ginger. Simmer 1 minute. Pour the hot sauce over the vegetables, sprinkle a little chopped parsley on top, and serve.

For a different flavor, puréed barley miso can be used to season this dish instead of shoyu. Use ¼–½ teaspoon per cup of liquid. Brown rice vinegar can also be added to provide a slightly sour taste. When all ingredients are cooked, add diluted miso and a tablespoon or so of vinegar, and serve.

*B*oiled Daikon with Black Sesame Seeds

3 cups daikon, sliced in ½-inch-thick
*   rounds*
pinch of sea salt
several lemon slices
black sesame seeds, washed and toasted
*   (see page 185)*
water

Place daikon in a pot. Add water to half cover daikon. Add a pinch of sea salt and bring to a boil. Cover, reduce flame to medium-low, and simmer 30–35 minutes, until daikon is tender. Remove daikon and place in a serving bowl or on a plate. Arrange several slices or half slices of fresh lemon around the edges of the serving bowl or plate and sprinkle a few toasted black sesame seeds on top of daikon rounds.

DAY 3

B R E A K F A S T   M E N U

❧

Whole Oats with Dulse Flakes

Toasted Rice Kayu Bread

Apple Butter

Bancha Tea or Grain Coffee
(see page 30)

Whole Oats with Dulse Flakes

1 cup whole oats, washed
5 cups water
pinch of sea salt
dulse flakes

Place washed oats and water in a pot. Add a pinch of sea salt. Bring to a boil. Cover and reduce flame to low. Place a flame deflector under the pot and leave to cook all night on a low flame. In the morning, place cereal in individual serving bowls and garnish each bowl with a small amount of dulse flakes.

If you do not want to cook this cereal overnight, first soak oats for 3–4 hours and then pressure-cook for 50 minutes. If pressure-cooking, be very careful not to have the flame too high, as there is a danger that the oats will foam up and clog the pressure vent.

Toasted Rice Kayu Bread

6–8 slices rice kayu bread

Toast rice kayu bread (see page 37) and serve with Apple Butter (below), or another spread.

Apple Butter

2 cups water or apple cider
pinch of sea salt
3 pounds apples, washed, peeled, cored,
*   and sliced*

Place water or cider, sea salt, and apples in a pot. Bring to a boil. Cover, reduce flame to medium-low, and simmer until apples are soft. Remove and purée in a hand food mill. Place apple purée back in pot. Simmer on a low flame, stirring occasionally, until apples become very thick and dark brown, and no liquid appears around the edges of the pot. Remove and use on your favorite bread, toast, or rice cakes. The proportions listed above yield approximately three-quarters of a pound. To store, allow to cool and place in a glass jar that can be tightly sealed. Apple butter will keep for about 2 weeks in the refrigerator.

Baked Tofu Sandwiches with Miso Spread

Boiled Watercress
(see page 65)

Bancha Tea
(see page 30)

*B*aked Tofu Sandwiches with Miso Spread

10 or 12 slices of tofu, 3 inches long by
* 2 inches wide by ¼–½ inch thick*
puréed barley miso
1 sheet toasted nori (see page 121)

Take 5 or 6 slices of tofu and spread a thin layer of puréed miso on each slice. Place the other slices on top of the miso layers to create 5 or 6 tofu sandwiches. Slice toasted nori into strips and wrap 1 strip around each sandwich. If necessary, use a little water to help the nori stick. Place nori-wrapped tofu sandwiches on a baking tray or dish. Bake at 350° F for 15–20 minutes. Remove and arrange on a serving platter or dish. Serve.

Brown Rice and Lotus Seeds

Miso Soup with Wakame and Scallions

Boiled Salad

Azuki, Chestnut, and Raisin Compote

Brown Rice and Lotus Seeds

2 cups brown rice, washed
1 cup lotus seeds, soaked 6–8 hours
2½–3 cups water
pinch of sea salt per cup of grain

Place brown rice and lotus seeds in a pressure cooker. Add water and place on a low flame for 15–20 minutes. Add sea salt. Turn flame to high and place cover on the cooker. Bring to pressure. Place a flame deflector under the cooker. Reduce flame to medium-low and cook for 50 minutes. After this time, remove from flame and bring the pressure down. Let rice sit for 4–5 minutes. Remove and serve in a wooden bowl.

Miso Soup with Wakame and Scallions

4–5 cups water
⅛ cup wakame, washed, soaked,
  and sliced
1½ tablespoons puréed barley miso
sliced scallions

Place water in a pot and bring to a boil. Add wakame. Cover, reduce flame to medium-low, and simmer 5–7 minutes or until wakame is soft. Turn flame to low and add puréed miso. Simmer 2–3 minutes and then place in individual serving bowls. Garnish each bowl with sliced scallions. Serve hot.

Boiled Salad

water
1 cup carrots, sliced into matchsticks
2 cups fresh cabbage
1 cup celery, sliced on a diagonal
1 cup sauerkraut (see page 157)
1 teaspoon chopped parsley
1 tablespoon toasted black sesame seeds

Place ½ inch of water in a pot and bring to a boil. Add carrots and boil for about 1 minute. Remove carrots and drain, reserving the cooking water. Place cabbage in the water from cooking carrots, and boil for about 1 minute. Stir cabbage around to cook evenly. Remove cabbage and drain, again reserving the cooking water. Place celery in the water from cooking carrots and cabbage and boil about 1 minute. Remove and drain. Mix carrots, cabbage, and celery together. Chop sauerkraut and mix it with cooked vegetables. Mix in chopped parsley.

To toast black sesame seeds, wash seeds, drain, and place in a dry skillet over medium-low flame. Stir constantly to prevent burning and shake pan occasionally to roast seeds evenly.

Seeds should be ready after about 5 minutes (they are done when they start to pop). Sprinkle toasted sesame seeds on top of salad vegetables for garnish, and serve.

$\mathcal{A}$zuki, Chestnut, and Raisin Compote

1 cup dried chestnuts, washed, dry-
roasted for 5–7 minutes, and then
soaked about 10–15 minutes
½–¾ cup raisins
1 cup azuki beans, soaked 6–8 hours
water
⅛–¼ teaspoon sea salt

Place chestnuts, raisins, and azuki beans in a heavy pot. Add just enough water to cover beans. Bring to a boil. Cover and reduce flame to medium-low. Simmer about 2–2½ hours. If necessary during this time, add water in small amounts only to just cover beans. After 2–2½ hours, season with a little sea salt. Continue to cook beans until most of the remaining liquid has cooked away. Place in individual serving dishes and serve.

This dessert is especially delicious served over hot, fresh mochi (page 50).

DAY 4

BREAKFAST MENU

❧

Soft Rice with Umeboshi

Chinese Cabbage Pickles

Bancha Tea or Grain Coffee

(see page 30)

Soft Rice with Umeboshi

1 cup brown rice
5 cups water
½–1 umeboshi plum
1 sheet nori
sliced scallions

Wash rice and place in pressure cooker. Add water and umeboshi. Cover pressure cooker, turn flame to medium-low, and bring up to pressure gradually. Place flame deflector under pot when pressure is up. Pressure-cook for 50 minutes. Remove from flame and allow pressure to come down. Remove cover when all pressure is out of the cooker, and place rice in individual serving bowls.

Toast a sheet of nori (see page 121) and cut it into thin strips about 2 inches long and ¼ inch wide. Garnish each bowl with scallion slices and several strips of nori. Serve hot.

Chinese Cabbage Pickles

2 cups Chinese cabbage
1–2 teaspoons sea salt

Slice cabbage very thin and place in a pickle press, crock, or bowl. Mix salt in with cabbage. Press with pressure plate of the pickle press or with a saucer and some kind of weight. Let sit several hours or overnight. If the pickles are too salty for your taste, simply rinse them before eating. Serve on a plate or in a bowl. This type of pickle will keep about 1 week if kept cool.

LUNCH MENU

Sprouted-Wheat Bread
with Amazake-Kuzu Sauce

Pickled Daikon Greens
(see page 44)

Grain Coffee
(see page 30)

Sprouted-Wheat Bread with Amazake-Kuzu Sauce

1 quart amazake
½ cup raisins, soaked
4–5 tablespoons kuzu, diluted in ⅓ cup
  cold water
8–10 slices sprouted wheat bread

Place amazake in a saucepan with raisins. Bring to a boil, cover, and reduce flame to medium-low. Simmer about 4–5 minutes. Reduce flame to low and add diluted kuzu, stirring constantly. When amazake becomes thick and creamy, remove and place in a serving bowl. Spoon this sauce over slices of sprouted-wheat bread.

DINNER MENU

Sweet Brown Rice and Chestnuts

Fried Tofu

Grated Daikon and Carrot

Watercress-Kuzu Soup

Hiziki with Konnyaku

Boiled Kale and Carrots

Sweet Brown Rice and Chestnuts

1 cup dried chestnuts
2 cups sweet brown rice
3¾–4½ cups water
pinch of sea salt per cup of grain
    and chestnuts

Wash chestnuts and dry-roast them in a skillet for several minutes. Stir constantly and keep the flame low to prevent burning. When through roasting the chestnuts, soak them with water to cover for about 10 minutes.

Wash rice and place in a pressure cooker. Add roasted chestnuts and fresh water. Place cooker on a low flame for 15–20 minutes. Add sea salt and cover. Turn flame to high and bring to pressure. When pressure is up, place a flame deflector under cooker and reduce flame to medium-low. Pressure-cook for 50 minutes. After this time, remove rice and chestnuts from flame and bring pressure down. Remove cover and let rice sit for 4–5 minutes. Serve in a wooden bowl.

Fried Tofu

dark sesame oil
10–12 slices fresh tofu, 3 inches long by
    2 inches wide by ½ inch thick
1 piece daikon root, 4–6 inches long
1 piece ginger, about 2 inches long
shoyu soy sauce

Place a small amount of dark sesame oil in a skillet and pan-fry tofu slices for 2–3 minutes on each side.

Grate about ½ cup fresh daikon, and place it in a small bowl. Grate about 2 tablespoons of fresh ginger and place in a small bowl. After placing 2 slices of fried tofu on each person's plate, garnish each serving with a pinch of grated ginger and a few drops of shoyu. Also serve a tablespoon of fresh grated daikon to each person.

Grated Daikon and Carrot

1 medium daikon
1 carrot, about 4 inches long
sliced scallions

Grate daikon and carrot on a flat grater. Arrange grated daikon in a serving bowl. Set grated carrot in the center of bowl. Do not mix. Garnish with scallion slices. Serve each person about 1 tablespoon or so of grated daikon and carrot.

Watercress-Kuzu Soup

2–3 shiitake mushrooms, soaked
1 strip kombu, 2 inches long, soaked
4–5 tablespoons kuzu
sea salt
4–5 cups water, including soaking water
*   from kombu and shiitake*
1 bunch watercress, washed

Soak shiitake for 15 minutes in 1 cup of water. Soak kombu for 5 minutes in ½ cup water. Place shiitake, shiitake soaking water, kombu, and kombu soaking water in a pot. Add additional water to make 4–5 cups of liquid, if necessary. Bring to a boil. Reduce flame to medium-low and cover. Simmer about 10 minutes. Remove shiitake and kombu and set aside for future use. Dilute kuzu in 4–5 tablespoons of water. Reduce flame under soup to low and add diluted kuzu. Stir constantly to prevent lumping. Season with a little sea salt and simmer about 3–5 minutes longer.

Wash watercress very well. Drop it into a separate pot of boiling water for about 30 seconds. Remove and drain.

Pour hot soup into individual serving bowls. Add 2–3 sprigs of cooked watercress to each bowl of soup. Serve hot.

Hiziki with Konnyaku

1 ounce hiziki (about 2 cups, soaked)
water
4 ounces konnyaku
1–1½ teaspoons dark sesame oil
shoyu soy sauce

Wash hiziki very quickly and soak for about 5 minutes. Reserve the soaking water. Place konnyaku in a saucepan with a little water and boil for 2–3 minutes. Remove konnyaku and rinse to remove strong smell. Discard the cooking water. Slice konnyaku into rectangles about 2½ inches long, ½ inch wide, and ⅛ inch thick. Slice soaked hiziki into ½-inch lengths. Heat 1–1½ teaspoons of dark sesame oil in a skillet. Sauté konnyaku for 3–4 minutes. Add hiziki and sauté for 3–4 minutes more. Add water to half cover hiziki and konnyaku. Bring to a boil. Reduce flame to medium-low. Simmer for about 45 minutes. Season with a little shoyu and continue to cook until almost all liquid is gone. Place in a serving bowl and serve.

Boiled Kale and Carrots

water
1 cup carrots, sliced on a diagonal
2 cups kale, sliced on a diagonal

Place about ½ inch of water in a pot and bring to a boil. Add carrots, cover, and boil for about 2–3 minutes. The carrots should be bright orange and remain slightly crisp when done. Remove and drain carrots, reserving the cooking water. Place carrots in a serving bowl. Place kale in the water from boiling the carrots and boil 2–3 minutes, moving kale around to cook evenly. When done, the kale should be bright green and slightly crisp. Remove kale, drain, and mix with boiled carrots. Serve.

DAY 5

BREAKFAST MENU

*Miso Soup with Wakame, Onions,
and Carrots*

Toasted Mochi
(see page 50)

Grated Daikon with Nori Strips

Bancha Tea or Grain Coffee
(see page 30)

Miso Soup with Wakame, Onions, and Carrots

1 cup onions, sliced in half-moons
½ cup carrots, sliced on a diagonal
⅛ cup wakame, soaked 3–5 minutes and sliced
4–5 cups water
½–1 teaspoon puréed barley miso per cup of water
sliced scallions

Place onions, carrots, and wakame in a pot. Add water and bring to a boil. Cover and reduce flame to medium-low. Simmer until carrots and onions are soft. Reduce flame to very low and add a small amount of puréed barley miso. Simmer 2–3 minutes. Place soup in individual serving bowls and garnish each bowl with a few scallion slices. Serve hot.

Grated Daikon with Nori Strips

1 piece daikon root, 4–6 inches long
  (½ cup freshly grated daikon)
1 sheet nori, toasted
  (see page 121)
shoyu soy sauce

Grate daikon. Cut toasted nori with a knife or pair of scissors into strips 2 inches long. Place 1 tablespoon of grated daikon on each serving plate. Place 1 or 2 drops of shoyu on each spoonful of daikon. Garnish with several strips of toasted nori. Serve with mochi.

LUNCH MENU

Sesame and Chestnut Ohagi

Boiled Kale
(see page 152)

Bancha Tea
(see page 30)

Sesame and Chestnut Ohagi

2 cups sweet brown rice
2½ cups water
pinch of sea salt per cup of rice

Wash sweet rice and place in a pressure cooker. Add water. Place on a low flame for 15–20 minutes. Add salt and cover. Bring to pressure and cook the same as for plain pressure-cooked rice (see page 46). When rice is cooked, place it in a heavy wooden bowl and pound it with a heavy wooden pestle or mallet especially made for pounding mochi or ohagi. If a mochi-pounding pestle is not available and you pound a very small amount of sweet rice, you can use the wooden pestle from a suribachi. Pound vigorously but in an orderly fashion for about 15–20 minutes. When you have finished pounding, take about 1 tablespoon of the dough at a time and roll it in or coat it with one or both of the coatings listed on page 74 (Chestnut Purée or Sesame Seed Topping) and form into the desired shape. Continue coating and shaping the dough until it is all used up.

Other coatings for ohagi can be made from azuki beans, sweet azuki beans, ground walnuts and tamari or miso, other kinds of nuts, gomashio, etc.

ᘒ

Fried Wheat and Rye

*Azuki Beans with Lotus Seeds
and Lotus Root*

Fu and Broccoli Soup

Dried Daikon and Shiitake

Boiled Chinese Cabbage

Apple Pie

ℱried Wheat and Rye

*1 cup whole-wheat berries, soaked
    6–8 hours*
¼ cup rye berries, soaked 6–8 hours
1½–2 cups water
pinch of sea salt
dark sesame oil
1 tablespoon chopped scallion root
½ cup onions, diced
¼ cup celery, diced
½ cup carrots, diced
shoyu soy sauce

Place wheat and rye berries in a pressure cooker with water and sea salt. Pressure-cook for 50 minutes. Remove and allow to cool. Heat a small amount of dark sesame oil in a skillet. Sauté scallion root and onion for 1–2 minutes. Add celery and carrots. Sauté 1 minute. Add cooked wheat and rye berries, sprinkle a little shoyu on top, and cover. Reduce flame to low. Cook until vegetables are tender. Season with a little more shoyu, if desired, and mix. Sauté 1–2 minutes more. Remove and place in a serving bowl. Serve while hot.

Azuki Beans with Lotus Seeds and Lotus Root

½ cup lotus seeds, washed and soaked
    6–8 hours
½ cup fresh lotus root, sliced in chunks
1 cup azuki beans, washed and soaked,
    6–8 hours
water
⅛ teaspoon sea salt
parsley sprig

Place lotus seeds and lotus root in a heavy pot. Place azuki beans on top of lotus root. Add enough water to almost cover azuki beans. Bring to a boil. Cover, reduce flame to medium-low, and simmer for about 2 hours. Add water as necessary while beans are cooking, only to almost cover. When beans are soft and tender, add ⅛ teaspoon of sea salt and continue to cook until most of the liquid has evaporated. The approximate cooking time is between 2 and 2½ hours. Place cooked beans in a serving bowl, garnish with a parsley sprig, and serve.

Fu and Broccoli Soup

1 piece kombu, 2 x 2 inches, soaked
4–5 cups water (including water from
    soaking fu)
1 cup fu, soaked 5–10 minutes in 2 cups
    of water, and sliced

1 cup broccoli florets
shoyu soy sauce

Place kombu and water in a pot and bring to a boil. Cover and reduce flame to medium-low. Simmer about 10 minutes. Remove kombu and set aside for future use. Add fu and simmer 5 minutes. Add broccoli. When broccoli is just about done, season with a little shoyu and simmer 1–2 minutes more. The broccoli should be bright green when done. Place in individual serving bowls and serve while hot.

Dried Daikon and Shiitake

3–4 shiitake mushrooms, soaked 10 min-
*   utes in 1 cup water, stems removed*
*   and sliced*
2 cups dried daikon, soaked 10 minutes
*   in water just to cover*
daikon and shiitake soaking water
shoyu soy sauce

Place shiitake in a pot. Set dried daikon on top. Add just enough soaking water to cover vegetables. Bring to a boil. Cover and reduce flame to low. Simmer 40–45 minutes or until very soft. Season with a little shoyu and simmer until almost all remaining liquid is gone. Place in a serving bowl and serve.

Boiled Chinese Cabbage

3 cups Chinese cabbage, sliced
water

Place about ½ inch of water in a pot. Add Chinese cabbage. Cook 2–3 minutes. Remove and drain. Place in a serving bowl and serve.

Apple Pie

pastry dough
10–12 baking apples, sliced
½ cup water
pinch of sea salt
¼ cup barley malt or brown rice syrup
2 tablespoon kuzu
¼–½ teaspoon cinnamon (optional)

Prepare a pie dough (see page 162) and roll out 2 crusts. Place one crust in a pie plate and press edges down with a fork. Poke several holes in the crust to prevent it from buckling while cooking. Prebake the empty bottom crust in a 350° F oven for about 10–15 minutes. While crust is baking, place apples, water, sea salt, and sweetener in a pot. Bring to a boil. Cover and reduce flame to medium-low. Cook until apples are done. Dilute kuzu with 2 tablespoons of water and add to apples, stirring constantly to prevent lumping. Simmer 2–3 minutes or just until kuzu thickens and becomes translucent. Remove and cool.

Place cooked apple filling inside shell. Place top crust over the apples and seal edges shut with a fork. Bake at 350° F for about 30 minutes or until top crust is golden brown and crisp. Remove pie and cool slightly before slicing.

DAY 6

BREAKFAST MENU

❦

Miso Soup with Wakame and Onions
(see page 56)

Scrambled Tofu

Onion-Shoyu Pickles
(see page 119)

Bancha Tea or Grain Coffee
(see page 30)

Scrambled Tofu

dark sesame oil
¼ cup burdock, sliced in matchsticks
1 cup onions, diced
½ cup carrots, sliced in matchsticks
2 cups cabbage, quartered and
*   finely sliced*
2 cakes (16 ounces each) tofu
umeboshi vinegar

Heat a small amount of dark sesame oil in a skillet. Sauté burdock 1–2 minutes. Add onions and carrots and sauté 1 minute. Add cabbage. Crumble tofu and set it on top of the vegetables. Cover and cook on a low flame for 3–4 minutes. Add several drops umeboshi vinegar and cook for 1–2 minutes more. The cooked vegetables should be bright in color and they should remain slightly crisp. Mix and place in a serving bowl. Serve.

Lunch Menu

☙

Vegetable Fried Whole-Wheat Spaghetti

Grain Coffee
(see page 30)

Vegetable Fried Whole-Wheat Spaghetti

8 ounces (dry weight) whole-wheat
  spaghetti
2 quarts water
dark sesame oil
1 cup carrots, sliced into matchsticks
1–2 tablespoons shoyu soy sauce
1 cup sliced scallions
1 tablespoon toasted sesame seeds

Boil spaghetti in water until done. To test for doneness, break a piece of spaghetti in half. The inside should be as dark as the outside. Remove, rinse under cold water, and drain. Heat a small amount of oil in a skillet. Add carrots and place spaghetti on top of them. Cover and reduce flame to low. Cook until carrots are almost tender. (In the summer months, it is best if they remain slightly crisp.) Add shoyu soy sauce and sliced scallions. Cover again and heat 2–3 more minutes. Mix cooked spaghetti and vegetables thoroughly and place in a serving dish. Mix toasted sesame seeds throughout, or sprinkle them on top, and serve.

DINNER MENU

☙

Brown Rice and Sesame Seeds

Oden

Sake Lees Miso Soup

Sautéed Cabbage, Kale, and Carrots

Rice Pudding

---

*B*rown Rice and Sesame Seeds

2 cups brown rice, washed
2½–3 cups water
pinch of sea salt per cup of rice
¼ cup roasted sesame seeds

Pressure-cook brown rice as previously instructed (see page 46). Remove cooked rice from pressure cooker and place in a bowl. Mix in roasted sesame seeds very well. Serve rice and sesame seeds in a serving bowl.

Oden

1 piece kombu, 2 x 2 inches, soaked
2 cups daikon, sliced into ½-inch-thick
*   rounds*
4–5 shiitake mushrooms, soaked, stems
*   removed, and sliced in half*
dark sesame oil
5–6 slices tofu, 2 inches by 3 inches by
*   ½-inch thick*
water
shoyu soy sauce

Soak kombu for 5 minutes in ½ cup water and slice into strips 3–4 inches long. Tie each strip into a bow, with a knot in the center. Place kombu bows in one section of a fairly large pot. Soak shiitake for 10 minutes in 1 cup water. Put daikon rounds next to kombu bows, and shiitake next to daikon.

Place a small amount of dark sesame oil in a skillet and lightly pan-fry each tofu slice on both sides.

Place fried tofu slices in the pot next to shiitake and kombu. Each ingredient should have a separate section of the pot; do not mix or layer the ingredients. Add water to half-cover the ingredients. Bring to a boil. Reduce flame to medium-low, cover, and simmer until daikon is soft and translucent. Season with a little shoyu and cook until there is only ¼ cup of liquid left. Place in a serving dish and serve.

Sake Lees Miso Soup

⅛ cup wakame, soaked 3 minutes and sliced
1 cup daikon, cut in matchsticks
4–5 cups water
3–4 teaspoons sake lees
2½–3½ teaspoons puréed barley miso

1 teaspoon fresh grated ginger
½ cup sliced scallions

Place wakame and daikon in a pot. Add water and bring to a boil. Cover and reduce flame to medium-low. Simmer until daikon is soft. Purée sake lees, add, and simmer 2–3 minutes. Add miso and simmer 2–3 additional minutes. Place soup in individual serving bowls. Add a pinch of ginger and about 1 teaspoon scallion to each bowl of soup. Serve hot.

Sautéed Cabbage, Kale, and Carrots

dark sesame oil
2 cups cabbage, sliced
pinch of sea salt
1 cup carrots, sliced in matchsticks
½ cup kale, chopped

Heat a small amount of dark sesame oil in a skillet. Maintain a high flame to keep vegetables crisp. Add cabbage and sea salt and sauté 1–2 minutes. Add carrots and kale and sauté 3–4 minutes more, constantly moving vegetables with a pair of chopsticks or a spoon to sauté evenly. The cooked vegetables should be crisp and bright colored. Place in a serving bowl and serve.

Rice Pudding

2 cups dried chestnuts
2 cups cooked brown rice
2 cups cooked sweet brown rice
1 cup chopped almonds
1 cup raisins
¼ teaspoon cinnamon (optional)
3½–4 cups apple juice

Dry-roast chestnuts in a skillet several minutes, stirring constantly to prevent burning. Remove chestnuts and soak covered with water for 10–15 minutes.

Place all ingredients including chestnuts in a pressure cooker and bring to pressure. Cook for 50 minutes. Remove from flame and bring pressure down. Remove cover and place pudding in a serving bowl. Serve hot.

DAY 7

BREAKFAST MENU

☙

Polenta with Parsley

Sauerkraut

Bancha Tea or Grain Coffee
(see page 30)

Polenta with Parsley

3 cups water
1 cup onion, diced
1 cup coarse ground polenta
pinch of sea salt per cup of polenta
¼ cup parsley, chopped

Place water in a pot and bring to a boil. Add diced onions, polenta, and a pinch of sea salt to the boiling water. Cover, reduce flame to medium-low, and simmer about 15 minutes. When done, mix in chopped parsley and place in individual serving bowls. Serve.

Sauerkraut

5 pounds cabbage
⅓ cup sea salt

Wash and finely shred cabbage. Place it in a wooden keg or ceramic crock. Mix sea salt in very well. Place several clean rocks or a heavy weight on top of a plate or wooden disk to press the cabbage. Cover keg or crock with a piece of clean cheesecloth or cotton linen to keep dust out. Within 10 hours the water level in the keg should be up to or above the plate. If the level is above the plate, remove some of the weight to make the water recede. Keep sauerkraut in a dark, cool place for about 1½ to 2 weeks. Check it every day to make sure all is going well. If mold begins to form on top, make sure to remove and discard it as soon as you notice it. If mold is not removed, it will cause the entire batch of sauerkraut to spoil.

Rinse sauerkraut with cold water and place 2–3 tablespoons on each individual serving plate or in bowls.

ↄ

Rice Croquettes

Shoyu-Ginger Sauce
(see page 152)

Boiled Cabbage

Bancha Tea
(see page 30)

*R*ice Croquettes

light sesame oil
8–10 cups cooked brown rice

Place about 2–3 inches of oil in a pot suitable for deep-frying. Heat oil, but do not let it get so hot that it smokes. Turn down flame to medium-low.

Form rice into firmly packed balls or triangles as you would when making rice balls (see page 71).

When the oil is hot, fry 2–3 balls of rice until golden brown, turning them occasionally to brown evenly. Remove and drain on clean paper towels. Repeat until all rice balls are fried. Serve with a spoonful or so of shoyu-ginger sauce over each croquette. The amount of rice given above should yield about 8–10 croquettes, or 2 per person.

Boiled Cabbage

water
3 cups cabbage, sliced
chopped parsley

Boil a small amount of water in a pot. Add cabbage, cover, and reduce flame to medium. Simmer 4 minutes or so. The cooked cabbage should be bright green and slightly crisp. Remove from water. Mix in chopped parsley and place in a serving bowl. Serve.

DINNER MENU

Pressure-Cooked White Rice

Sweet and Sour Seitan

Grated Daikon with Sliced Scallions

Boiled Chinese Cabbage and Kale

Apricot Couscous Cake

Pressure-Cooked White Rice

2 cups organic white sushi rice
pinch of sea salt
2½ cups water

Place rice, sea salt and water in a pressure cooker. Cover and bring to pressure. Reduce flame to low. Cook 15 minutes. Remove and allow pressure to come down. Remove rice and place in a bowl.

Sweet and Sour Seitan

2 cups cooked seitan (see page 158), sliced
1 cup burdock, sliced in chunks
1 cup apple juice
3 cups seitan-shoyu cooking water (see page 158)
3–4 tablespoons kuzu, diluted in 3 to 4 tablespoons water
small amount of brown rice vinegar
¼ cup chopped scallions

Place seitan, burdock, apple juice, and seitan-shoyu cooking water in a pot. Bring to a boil. Cover and reduce flame to medium-low. Simmer 5–7 minutes, until burdock is soft. Reduce flame to low and add diluted kuzu and a small amount of brown rice vinegar. Simmer 2–3 minutes. When done, place in a serving bowl and mix in chopped scallions. Serve hot.

Grated Daikon with Sliced Scallions

1 cup grated daikon
shoyu soy sauce
sliced scallions

Place grated daikon in a serving bowl. Pour several drops of shoyu in the middle of the daikon. Garnish with a few scallion slices. Serve.

When served, each person can take a tablespoon of daikon and eat it with 1 or 2 drops of shoyu.

*B*oiled Chinese Cabbage and Kale

2 cups Chinese cabbage, sliced
1 cup kale, sliced
water

Place about one-half inch of water in a pot and bring to a boil. Add Chinese cabbage, cover, and simmer 2–3 minutes. Remove cabbage, and drain it, but keep the boiling water. Place cabbage in a serving dish. Drop kale in the pot of boiling water and boil 2–3 minutes. Remove and drain. Mix kale with Chinese cabbage or arrange it around the outside of the Chinese cabbage to form a ring effect, and serve.

*A*pricot Couscous Cake

2 cups couscous
2½ cups apple juice or water
½ cup raisins
pinch of sea salt

Wash couscous and drain. Place apple juice or water in a pot. Add raisins and sea salt and bring to a boil. Cover and reduce flame to medium-low. Simmer about 10 minutes. Add couscous. Cover and simmer 2–3 minutes. Turn off flame and let couscous sit covered for several minutes. (The heat in the pot will cause the couscous to cook thoroughly.) Remove and place couscous in a glass or ceramic cake dish. Press couscous down firmly with a rice paddle before adding topping.

TOPPING
2 cups dried apricots
pinch of sea salt
2 cups water
4–5 tablespoons kuzu diluted in water
1 lemon slice

Place dried apricots in a pressure cooker. Add a pinch of sea salt and 2 cups of water. Cover and bring to pressure. Pressure-cook about 15–20 minutes. Bring pressure down and remove cover. Purée apricots and put them back in cooker. Dilute kuzu. Place cooker on a low flame and add diluted kuzu, stirring constantly to prevent lumping. Simmer until apricot mixture becomes thick. Remove and cool slightly.

Spread apricot mixture evenly to cover couscous cake. Garnish with a lemon slice. Allow cake to sit for about 1 hour before slicing and serving.

Changing Seasons Menu Guide

In this book, over a hundred basic dishes are presented. These dishes represent only a fraction of the thousands of combinations and variations used in macrobiotic cooking. As you can see, rather than limiting your dietary options, the macrobiotic diet widens them considerably.

For your convenience in choosing the dishes you wish to prepare, the following Menu Guide lists the menus in the order in which they appear in the text.

As mention previously, feel free to change, modify, or elaborate on the menus or recipes, or to prepare them in any order that you like. It is important to be flexible and to adapt your cooking to your individual needs. Change and creativity are essential ingredients in macrobiotic cooking.

SPRING

	BREAKFAST	LUNCH	DINNER
DAY 1	Soft Rice with Umeboshi Broccoli and Cauliflower 　Shoyu Pickles Bancha Tea or Grain 　Coffee	Vegetable Fried Soba 　Noodles Grain Coffee	Rice and Black Beans Steamed Tempeh and 　Sauerkraut Miso Soup with Wakame 　and Daikon Boiled Salad with Sauce Applesauce Barley Tea
DAY 2	Oatmeal Onion Butter Rice Kayu Bread Bancha Tea or Grain 　Coffee	Boiled Buckwheat and 　Vegetables Bancha Tea	Brown Rice and Wheat 　Berries Lentil Soup Steamed Kale and 　Carrots Whole Onions and Miso 　with Parsley Plum Tarts or Stewed 　Plums
DAY 3	Miso Soft Rice Pickled Daikon or Turnip 　Greens Bancha Tea or Grain 　Coffee	Fried Tofu Sandwiches 　with Mustard Grain Coffee	Pressure-Cooked Brown 　Rice Creamy Barley Soup Fried Soba Tempeh Cabbage Rolls Arame with Onions Apple-Pear-Raisin Kuzu 　Sauce

	BREAKFAST	LUNCH	DINNER
DAY 4	Toasted Mochi Grated Daikon with Nori Strips Bancha Tea or Grain Coffee	Peanut Butter and Apple Cider Jelly Sandwiches Dill Pickles Bancha Tea	Nishime Vegetables Fried Rice with Wild Vegetables Clear Soup Chick Peas with Carrots Boiled Mustard Greens
DAY 5	Miso Soup with Wakame and Onions Toasted Bread with Apple Butter Steamed Broccoli Bancha Tea or Grain Coffee	Rice Balls with Umeboshi Boiled Vegetable Salad Grain Coffee	Millet with Almonds Baked Tofu with Miso Sauce Carrot Soup Chinese Cabbage with Shoyu-Lemon Sauce Macro-Jacks
DAY 6	Creamy Rice with Kamut Steamed Tempeh, Sauerkraut, and Cabbage Bancha Tea or Grain Coffee	Deep-Fried Millet Croquettes Grated Daikon Boiled Watercress Bancha Tea	Brown Rice with Shiso Leaves Azuki Beans with Wheat Berries Clear Shoyu-Watercress Soup Kale with Sour Tofu Dressing Chinese-Style Vegetables with Kuzu Sauce Baked Stuffed Apples

	BREAKFAST	LUNCH	DINNER
DAY 7	Miso Soup with Wakame, Onions, and Tofu Rice Balls Bancha Tea or Grain Coffee	Steamed Leftover Rice Sautéed Tofu and Vegetables Grain Coffee	Sesame and Chestnut Ohagi Clear Broth Kimpira Burdock, Carrot, and Dried Tofu Boiled Cauliflower and Broccoli with Shoyu Ginger-Lemon Sauce

SUMMER

	BREAKFAST	LUNCH	DINNER
DAY 1	Miso Soup with Wakame and Daikon Boiled Tofu with Ginger-Parsley Sauce Bancha Tea or Grain Coffee	Vegetable Fried Whole-Wheat Spaghetti Bancha Tea	Brown Rice and Spelt Boiled String Beans with Almonds Cool Chick Pea Soup Hiziki Salad with Tofu Dressing Strawberry Couscous Cake
DAY 2	Soft Millet with Green Nori Flakes Condiment Rutabaga-Shoyu Pickles Bancha Tea or Grain Coffee	Udon with Cool Broth and Nori Garnish Grain Coffee	Long-Grain Brown Rice with Fresh Corn Japanese Black Soy Beans Miso Soup with Wakame and Daikon Chinese-Style Sautéed Vegetables with Sauce Fresh Watermelon

	BREAKFAST	LUNCH	DINNER

DAY 3	Soft Rice and Barley
	Broiled Tofu
	Bancha Tea or Grain
	  Coffee
		Sautéed Seitan Slices with
		  Onions and Mustard
		Corn on the Cob with
		  Umeboshi
		Bancha Tea
			Buckwheat Salad
			Lentils
			Clear Soup with Tofu
			  and Watercress
			Baked Summer Squash
			  with Miso-Ginger
			  Sauce
			Boiled Carrots and
			  Burdock
			Cool Amazake Cherry
			  Pudding

DAY 4	Soft Barley with Scallions
	  and Nori Strips
	Red Radish Pickles
	Bancha Tea or Grain
	  Coffee
		Seitan Sandwiches with
		  Lettuce and Cucumber
		  Slices
		Grain Coffee
			Boiled Rice
			Scrambled Tofu and
			  Corn
			Miso Soup with Fu
			Sautéed Chinese Cabbage
			  and Snow Peas
			Blueberry Pie

DAY 5	Miso Soup with Wakame,
	  Carrots, and Broccoli
	Toasted Mochi
	Grated Daikon with Nori
	  Strips
	Bancha Tea or Grain
	  Coffee
		Cucumber-Rice Sushi
		Bancha Tea
			Millet and Sweet Corn
			Kidney Beans
			Cauliflower Soup
			Arame with Tempeh and
			  Onions
			Steamed Kale
			Fruit Salad

	BREAKFAST	LUNCH	DINNER
DAY 6	Buckwheat Pancakes with Apple-Raisin-Kuzu Sauce Chinese Cabbage Pickles Bancha Tea or Grain Coffee	Baked Corn on the Cob with Ginger-Shoya Sauce Whole-Wheat or Rice Kayu Bread Onion Butter Grain Coffee	Brown Rice and Lotus Seeds Dried Tofu, Carrots, and Onions Whole-Wheat Somen and Broth Boiled Cabbage Cherry Strudel
DAY 7	Soft Millet and Sweet Corn Onion-Shoyu Pickles Bancha Tea or Grain Coffee	Somen with Cool Broth Boiled Watercress Garnish Toasted Nori Strips Bancha Tea	Brown Rice Salad Azuki Beans Miso Soup with Tofu Arame with Sweet Corn and Onions Boiled Turnip Greens with Sesame Seeds Fresh Cantaloupe Slices

AUTUMN

	BREAKFAST	LUNCH	DINNER
DAY 1	Soft Rice with Squash Turnip-Kombu Pickles Bancha Tea or Grain Coffee	Rice Balls Rolled in Toasted Sesame Seeds Vegetable Salad with Vinegar-Ginger-Shoyu Sauce Grain Coffee	Boiled Barley Soybean Stew Chinese Cabbage Pickles Peach Crunch

	BREAKFAST	LUNCH	DINNER
DAY 2	Soft Rice with Umeboshi Steamed Kale Bancha Tea or Grain Coffee	Tempeh Sandwiches Bancha Tea	Millet with Squash Yu-Dofu Miso Soup with Deep- Fried Croutons Kimpira Carrots and Burdock Arame with Lotus Root Amazake Pudding
DAY 3	Miso Soup with Squash Skins Boiled Tempeh Bancha Tea or Grain Coffee	Millet and Squash Stew Chinese Cabbage Pickles Grain Coffee	Brown Rice with Wild Rice Puréed Squash Soup Chinese-Style Sautéed Vegetables Kombu Carrot Rolls Kidney Beans with Miso
DAY 4	Miso Soup with Wakame and Daikon Broiled Tofu Bancha Tea or Grain Coffee	Fried Wild Rice with Tofu and Vegetables Pickled Daikon or Turnip Greens Bancha Tea	Azuki Beans and Squash Cauliflower Clear Soup Steamed or Boiled Kale Baked Apples with Kuzu- Raisin Sauce
DAY 5	Soft Millet with Corn and Onions Onion-Shoyu Pickles Bancha Tea or Grain Coffee	Pan-Fried Rice Croquettes Shoyu-Ginger Sauce Boiled Kale Grain Coffee	Sweet Brown Rice and Azuki Beans Deep-Fried Tofu with Kuzu Sauce Daikon Clear Soup Celery, Carrot, Apple, and Dulse Salad Steamed Kale

	BREAKFAST	LUNCH	DINNER
DAY 6	Soft Bulgur with Scallions Sauerkraut Bancha Tea or Grain Coffee	Boiled Seitan Steamed Cabbage Bancha Tea	Millet and Vegetables Goma Wakame Condiment Creamy Barley Soup Nishime Vegetables with Tofu Sautéed Bok Choy Squash Pie
DAY 7	Miso Soup with Wakame and Cauliflower Toasted Sourdough Bread Carrot Butter Bancha Tea or Grain Coffee	Steamed Mochi and Chinese Cabbage Sautéed Vegetables Grain Coffee	Brown Rice Seitan Squash Stew Arame with Lotus Seeds Steamed Collard Greens

WINTER

	BREAKFAST	LUNCH	DINNER
DAY 1	Miso Soup with Wakame and Daikon Boiled Tofu, Broccoli, and Carrots Bancha Tea or Grain Coffee	Boiled Fu with Tofu, Broccoli, and Carrots Bancha Tea	Brown Rice and Azuki Beans Seitan Barley Stew Arame with Dried Tofu and Carrots Boiled Collard Greens

	BREAKFAST	LUNCH	DINNER
DAY 2	Miso Soft Rice Pickled Mustard Greens Bancha Tea or Grain Coffee	Rice and Azuki Bean Stew Sautéed Chinese Cabbage Grain Coffee	Gomoku Tempeh and Onions with Kuzu-Ginger Sauce Boiled Daikon with Black Sesame Seeds Boiled Watercress
DAY 3	Whole Oats with Dulse Flakes Toasted Rice Kayu Bread Apple Butter Bancha Tea or Grain Coffee	Baked Tofu Sandwiches with Miso Spread Boiled Watercress Bancha Tea	Brown Rice and Lotus Seeds Miso Soup with Wakame and Scallions Boiled Salad Azuki, Chestnut, and Raisin Compote
DAY 4	Soft Rice with Umeboshi Chinese Cabbage Pickles Bancha Tea or Grain Coffee	Sprouted-Wheat Bread with Amazake-Kuzu Sauce Pickled Daikon Greens Grain Coffee	Sweet Brown Rice and Chestnuts Fried Tofu Grated Daikon and Carrot Watercress-Kuzu Soup Hiziki with Konnyaku Boiled Kale and Carrots
DAY 5	Miso Soup with Wakame, Onions, and Carrots Toasted Mochi Grated Daikon with Nori Strips Bancha Tea or Grain Coffee	Sesame and Chestnut Ohagi Boiled Kale Bancha Tea	Fried Wheat and Rye Azuki Beans with Lotus Seeds and Lotus Root Fu and Broccoli Soup Dried Daikon and Shiitake Boiled Chinese Cabbage Apple Pie

	BREAKFAST	LUNCH	DINNER
DAY 6	Miso Soup with Wakame and Onions Scrambled Tofu Onion-Shoyu Pickles Bancha Tea or Grain Coffee	Vegetable Fried Whole-Wheat Spaghetti Grain Coffee	Brown Rice and Sesame Seeds Oden Sake Lees Miso Soup Sautéed Cabbage, Kale, and Carrots Rice Pudding
DAY 7	Polenta with Parsley Sauerkraut Bancha Tea or Grain Coffee	Rice Croquettes Shoyu-Ginger Sauce Boiled Cabbage Bancha Tea	Pressure-Cooked White Rice Sweet and Sour Seitan Grated Daikon with Sliced Scallions Boiled Chinese Cabbage and Kale Apricot Couscous Cake

RECOMMENDED READING

Books

Aihara, Cornellia. *The Do of Cooking.* Chico, Calif.: George Ohsawa Macrobiotic Foundation, 1972.

Brown, Virginia, with Susan Stayman. *Macrobiotic Miracle: How a Vermont Family Overcame Cancer.* New York: Japan Publications, 1984.

Dietary Goals for the United States. Washington, D.C.: Select Committee on Nutrition and Human Needs, U.S. Senate, 1977.

Diet, Nutrition, and Cancer. Washington, D.C.: National Academy of Sciences, 1982.

Dufty, William. *Sugar Blues.* New York: Warner, 1975.

East West Foundation. *Cancer and Heart Disease: The Macrobiotic Approach to Degenerative Disorders.* New York: Japan Publications, 1982.

Esko, Edward, and Wendy Esko. *Macrobiotic Cooking for Everyone.* New York: Japan Publications, 1980.

Esko, Wendy. *Introducing Macrobiotic Cooking.* New York: Japan Publications, 1978.

Fukuoaka, Masanobu. *The One-Straw Revolution.* Emmaus, Pa.: Rodale Press, 1978.

Healthy People: The Surgeon General's Report on Health Promotion and Disease Prevention. Washington, D.C.: Government Printing Office, 1979.

Heidenry, Carolyn. *An Introduction to Macrobiotics.* Brooklyn, Mass.: Alladin Press, 1984.

Hippocrates. *Hippocratic Writings.* Edited by G. E. R. Lloyd. Translated by J. Chadwick and W. N. Mann. New York: Penguin, 1978.

I Ching or Book of Changes. Translated by Richard Wilhelm and Cary F. Baynes. Princeton: Bollingen Foundation, 1950.

Jacobson, Michael. *The Changing American Diet.* Washington, D.C.: Center for Science in the Public Interest, 1978.

Kohler, Jean, and Mary Alice Kohler. *Healing Miracles from Macrobiotics.* West Nyack, N.Y.: Parker, 1979.

Kushi, Aveline. *How to Cook with Miso.* New York: Japan Publications, 1978.

———. *Lessons of Night and Day.* Wayne, N.J.: Avery, 1984.

Kushi, Aveline, with Alex Jack. *The Complete Macrobiotic Cookbook: Cooking for Health, Harmony, and Peace.* New York: Warner, 1985.

Kushi, Michio. *The Book of Do-In: Exercise for Physical and Spiritual Development.* New York: Japan Publications, 1979.

———. *The Book of Macrobiotics.* New York: Japan Publications, 1977.

———. *The Era of Humanity.* Brookline, Mass.: East West Journal, 1980.

———. *How to See Your Health: The Book of Oriental Diagnosis.* New York: Japan Publications, 1980.

———. *Macrobiotics: Experience the Miracle of Life.* Edited by Edward Esko. Brookline, Mass.: East West Foundation, 1978.

———. *Natural Healing through Macrobiotics.* New York: Japan Publications, 1978.

———. *On the Greater Life: Collected Thoughts and Ideas of Michio Kushi on Macrobiotics and Humanity.* Wayne, N.J.: Avery, 1985.

———. *Your Face Never Lies.* Wayne, N.J.: Avery, 1983.

Kushi, Michio, and Alex Jack. *The Cancer-Prevention Diet.* New York: St. Martin's, 1983.

Kushi, Michio and Aveline. *Macrobiotic Pregnancy and Care of the Newborn.* Edited by Edward and Wendy Esko. New York: Japan Publications, 1983.

Kushi, Michio, and the East West Foundation. *The Macrobiotic Approach to Cancer.* Wayne, N.J.: Avery, 1982.

Mendelsohn, Robert S., M.D. *Confessions of a Medical Heretic.* Chicago: Contemporary Books, 1979.

———. *Male Practice.* Chicago: Contemporary Books, 1980.

Ohsawa, George. *Cancer and the Philosophy of the Far East.* Oroville, Calif.: George Ohsawa Macrobiotic Foundation, 1971 edition.

————. *You Are All Sanpaku.* Edited by William Dufty. New York: University Books, 1965.

————. *Zen Macrobiotics.* Los Angeles: Ohsawa Foundation, 1965.

Price, Weston A., D.D.S. *Nutrition and Physical Degeneration.* Santa Monica, Calif.: Price-Pottenger Nutrition Foundation, 1945.

Sattilaro, Anthony, M.D., with Tom Monte. *Recalled by Life: The Story of My Recovery from Cancer.* Boston: Houghton-Mifflin, 1982.

Tara, William. *Macrobiotics and Human Behavior.* New York: Japan Publications, 1984.

Yamamoto, Shizuko. *Barefoot Shiatsu.* New York: Japan Publications, 1979.

The Yellow Emperor's Classic of Internal Medicine. Translated by Ilza Veith. Berkeley: University of California Press, 1949.

PERIODICALS

Macromuse, Washington, D.C.

Nutrition Action, Washington, D.C.

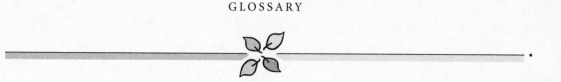

Aduki. *See* Azuki Bean.

Agar-agar. A white gelatin derived from a sea vegetable, used in making kanten and aspics. Kanten is excellent in the summer as a cool, refreshing dessert.

Albi. *See* Taro.

Amazake. A sweetener or refreshing drink made from rice or sweet rice and koji starter that is allowed to ferment into a thick liquid. Hot amazake is a delicious sweet beverage on cold autumn or winter nights.

Arame. A thin, wiry black sea vegetable similar to hiziki, often used as a side dish. Arame is rich in iron, calcium, and other minerals.

Arrowroot. A starch flour processed from the root of an American native plant. It is used as a thickening agent, similar to cornstarch or kuzu, for making sauces, stews, gravies, or desserts.

Azuki Bean. A small, dark red bean imported from Japan, but also grown in this country. Especially good when cooked with kombu sea vegetable. This bean may also be referred to as *aduki* or *adzuki*.

Bancha Tea. Correctly named *kukicha,* bancha consists of the stems and leaves from mature Japanese tea bushes. This tea aids in digestion and contains no chemical dyes. Bancha makes an excellent breakfast or after-dinner beverage.

Barley Malt. A thick, dark brown sweetener made from barley or a combination of barley and corn. Used in making desserts, sweet and sour sauces, and in a variety of medicinal drinks.

Barley, Pearl. A particular strain of barley native to China, pearl barley grows easily in colder climates. It is good in stews and mixed with other grains such as rice. It is effective in breaking down animal fats in the body.

Beefsteak Plant. *See* Shiso.

Black Sesame Seeds. Small black seeds, occasionally used as a garnish or in black gomashio, a condiment. A different variety of seed from the usual white or blond sesame seeds.

Bok Choy. A leafy, green vegetable used mostly in summer cooking. Available in many natural-food stores or Oriental grocery stores. Sometimes called *pok choy.*

Brown Rice. Whole, unpolished rice. It comes in three main varieties: short, medium, and long grain and contains an ideal balance of minerals, protein, and carbohydrates.

Brown Rice Vinegar. A very mild, delicate vinegar made from fermented brown rice or sweet brown rice. Not as sour as apple cider vinegar.

Buckwheat. Eaten as a staple food in many European countries, this cereal plant is eaten widely in the forms of kasha, whole groats, and soba noodles.

Burdock. A hardy plant that grows wild throughout the United States. The long, dark burdock root is delicious in soups, stews, and sea vegetable dishes, or sautéed with carrots. It is highly valued in macrobiotic cooking for its strengthening qualities. The Japanese name is *gobo.*

Chinese Cabbage. A large, leafy vegetable with pale green leaves at the top and thick, white leaves at the stem. It is often called *nappa,* and is juicy and somewhat sweet tasting. Good in soups and stews, vegetable dishes, and as a pickle.

Daikon. A long, white radish. Besides making a delicious side dish, daikon is a specific aid in dissolving fat and mucous deposits that have accumulated as a result of past animal food intake. Grated daikon aids in the digestion of oily foods.

Dried Daikon. Many natural-food stores now carry packaged daikon that has been shredded and dried. This is especially good cooked with kombu and seasoned with a little shoyu. Soaking dried daikon before use brings out its natural sweetness.

Dried Tofu. Tofu that has been naturally dehydrated by freezing. Used in soups, stews, vegetable, and sea vegetable dishes. Less fatty than regular tofu. *See also* Tofu.

Dulse. A reddish purple sea vegetable used in soups, salads, and vegetable dishes. Very high in protein, vitamin A, iodine, and phosphorus. Used for centuries in European cooking, dulse is now harvested on both sides of the North Atlantic (including off the coasts of Maine and Massachusetts).

Fu. A dried wheat gluten product. Available in thin sheets or thick, round cakes. Used in soups, stews, and vegetable dishes. High in protein.

Ginger. A spicy, pungent, golden-colored root, used as a garnish or seasoning in cooking. Also used in making external home remedies such as the ginger compress.

Gluten (Wheat). The sticky substance that remains after the bran has been kneaded and rinsed from whole-wheat flour. Used to make seitan and fu.

Gobo. *See* Burdock.

Gomashio. A condiment made from roasted, ground sesame seeds and sea salt. Gomashio is a rich source of minerals and whole oil and can be sprinkled lightly on rice and other grains.

Goma Wakame Powder. A condiment made from roasted and crushed wakame and sesame seeds. Also rich in minerals and other essential nutrients. Used like gomashio.

Gomoku. A dish made by combining a variety of grains and beans. Traditionally made from a combination of four whole grains and one variety of beans, this hearty dish is used primarily in fall and winter.

Grain Coffee. A noncaffeine coffee substitute made from roasted grains, beans, and roots. Ingredients are combined in different ways to create a variety of flavors. Used like instant coffee.

Green Nori Flakes. A sea vegetable condiment made from a certain type of nori, different from the packaged variety. The flakes are rich in iron, calcium, and vitamin A. Can be sprinkled on whole grains, vegetables, salads, and other dishes.

Hiziki. A dark brown sea vegetable that turns black when dried. It has a wiry consistency and may be strong tasting. Hiziki imported from Japan or harvested off the coast of Maine is available dried and packaged in most natural-food stores. It is very high in calcium and protein. Also known as hijiki.

Hokkaido Pumpkin. There are two varieties of Hokkaido pumpkin. One has a deep orange color and the other has a light green skin similar to Hubbard squash. Hokkaido pumpkins are available at many natural-food stores and by mail order. They have a tough outer skin and are very sweet inside.

Japanese Black Beans. A special type of soybean grown in Japan. It may be used medicinally to treat reproductive problems. In cooking, black beans are used in soups and side dishes.

Kampyo. Dried gourd strips that are first soaked and then used to bind vegetable rolls. The kampyo can be eaten along with the vegetable rolls.

Kanten. A jelled dessert made from agar-agar. It can include melon, apples, berries, peaches, pears, amazake, azuki beans, or other items. Usually served chilled, it is a cool refreshing alternative to conventional gelatin.

Kayu. Cereal grain that has been cooked with approximately five to ten times as much water as grain for a long period of time. Kayu is ready when it is soft and creamy.

Kimpira. A sautéed burdock or burdock-and-carrot dish that is seasoned with shoyu. This hearty root vegetable dish, used most often in fall and winter, imparts strength and vitality.

Kombu. A wide, thick, dark green sea vegetable that grows in deep ocean water. Often cooked with vegetables and beans, and used in making condiments, candy, and soup stocks. A single strip of kombu may be reused several times to flavor soups. Kombu is rich in essential minerals. Scientific research has discovered that it is effective in helping to prevent a variety of cancers.

Konnyaku. A gelatinous mold made in Japan from wild mountain potatoes. There are several varieties; all must be boiled and rinsed to remove their strong bitter taste before they are added to other dishes. Used in sea vegetable and nishime dishes.

Kudzu. *See* Kuzu.

Kukicha. *See* Bancha Tea.

Kuzu. A white starch made from the root of the wild kuzu plant. In this country, the plant is often called *kudzu*. Used in making soups, sauces, gravies, desserts, and for medicinal purposes.

Lotus. The root and seeds of a water lily that is brown skinned with a hollow, chambered, off-white inside. Especially good for the respiratory organs. The seeds are used in grain, bean, and sea vegetable dishes.

Millet. This small, yellow grain, which comes in many varieties, can be eaten on a regular basis. It can be used in soups, vegetable dishes, or eaten as a cereal.

Mirin. A wine made from whole-grain sweet rice. Used occasionally as a seasoning in vegetable or sea vegetable dishes.

Miso. A fermented grain or bean paste made from ingredients such as soybeans, barley, and rice. There are many varieties of miso now available. Barley (mugi) or soybean (hatcho) miso is usually recommended for daily use. The recipes in this book call for mugi miso fermented for several years. Miso is high in protein and vitamin B_{12}. It is especially good for the circulatory and digestive organs.

Miso, Puréed. Miso that has been reduced to a texture that will allow it to blend easily with other ingredients. To purée miso, place it in a bowl or suribachi and add enough water or broth to make a smooth paste. Blend with a wooden pestle or spoon.

Mochi. A rice cake or dumpling made from cooked, pounded sweet rice. In Japan, where mochi was first developed, it is traditionally eaten on New Year's day. Mochi is especially good for lactating mothers, as it promotes the production of breast milk.

Mugicha. A tea made from roasted, unhulled barley and water. It can be served chilled in summer.

Nappa. *See* Chinese Cabbage.

Natto. Soybeans that have been cooked and mixed with beneficial enzymes and allowed to ferment for twenty-four hours under a controlled temperature.

Nishime. A method of cooking in which different combinations of vegetables, sea vegetables, or soybean products are simmered for a long time over a low flame. Nishime is seasoned with shoyu or miso, and cooked until almost all the water in the pot is gone. The ingredients become soft, sweet, and easily digested. Also referred to as *waterless cooking*.

Nori. Thin sheets of dried sea vegetable that are black or dark purple when dried. Nori is often roasted over a flame until green. It is used as a garnish, wrapped around rice balls in making sushi, or cooked with tamari as a condiment. Rich in Vitamin A and protein, nori also contains calcium, iron, and vitamins B_1, B_2, C, and D.

Oden. A special dish in which root vegetables, sea vegetables, soybean products, and sometimes fish are simmered together for a long time. Many combinations of ingredients are used. This thick stew is good on cold winter nights.

Ohagi. Glutinous patties made from cooked, pounded sweet rice rolled in or coated with roasted and ground sesame seeds; roasted, ground, and shoyu-seasoned walnuts; cooked and puréed azuki beans or azuki beans and raisins; cooked and puréed dried chestnuts; or roasted soybean flour and rice honey. Ohagi may be eaten as a dessert.

Pok Choy. *See* Bok Choy.

Pressed Salad. Very thinly sliced or shredded fresh vegetables, combined with a pickling agent such as sea salt, umeboshi, grain vinegar, or shoyu, and placed in a special pickle press. In the pickling process, many of the enzymes and vitamins are retained while the vegetables become easier to digest.

Rice Balls. Rice shaped into balls or triangles, usually with a piece of umeboshi in the center, and wrapped in toasted nori or shiso leaves to completely cover. Pickles, seeds, vegetables, fried tofu, and other ingredients can be placed in the center to create a variety of tastes. Rice balls can also be coated with whole or ground sesame seeds. Good for snacks, lunches, picnics, and traveling.

Sake Lees. Fermented residue from making sake (rice wine). Used now and then as a seasoning in soups, stews, vegetable dishes, and pickles. Sake lees is especially good in the winter, as it tends to generate heat.

Sea Salt. Salt obtained from evaporated sea water, as opposed to rock salt. It is either sun baked or kiln baked. High in trace minerals, it contains no harmful chemicals, sugar, or iodine.

Seitan. Wheat gluten cooked in shoyu, kombu, and water. Seitan can be made at home or purchased ready-made at many natural-food stores. Many people use it as a meat substitute.

Sesame Butter. A nut butter obtained by roasting and grinding sesame seeds until smooth and creamy. Used like peanut butter or in salad dressings and sauces.

Shiitake Mushrooms. Dried shiitake are imported from Japan. Fresh shiitake, grown in this country, have recently come on the market. Either type can be used in soup stocks or vegetable dishes, and dried shiitake are used in medicinal preparations. These mushrooms are effective in helping the body to discharge excess salt and animal fats.

Shio Kombu. Pieces of kombu cooked for a long time in shoyu and used as a condiment. Use only a few pieces at a time, as shio kombu has a strong salty taste.

Shio Nori. Pieces of nori cooked for a long time in shoyu and water. Used occasionally as a condiment, shio nori is particularly tasty as a relish.

Shiso. A red, pickled leaf. The plant is known in English as the *beefsteak plant*. It is used to color umeboshi plums and as a condiment. Sometimes called *chiso*.

Shoyu. A naturally fermented soy sauce, made from soybeans with barley or wheat.

Soba. Noodles made from buckwheat flour or a combination of buckwheat with whole-wheat flour. Can be served in broth, in salads, or chilled in the summer. Eaten widely in Japan.

Somen. Very thin, white, or whole-wheat Japanese noodles. Often served during the summer. Somen are thinner than soba and other whole-grain noodles.

Sprouted-Wheat Bread. A whole-grain bread made from soaked wheat that is sprouted and baked. It does not contain flour and is very sweet and moist.

Suribachi. A special serrated, glazed clay bowl. Used with a pestle, called a surikogi, for grinding and puréeing foods. An essential item in a macrobiotic kitchen, the suribachi can be used in a variety of ways to make condiments, spreads, dressings, baby foods, nut butters, and medicinal preparations.

Surikogi. A wooden pestle that is used with a suribachi. Used to make gomashio, sea vegetable powders, and other condiments and to mash foods to obtain a creamy consistency.

Sushi. Rice rolled with vegetables, fish, or pickles, wrapped in nori, and sliced in rounds. Sushi is becoming increasingly popular throughout the United States. The best-quality sushi is made with brown rice and other natural ingredients.

Sushi Mat. Very thin strips of bamboo that are fastened together with cotton thread so that they can be rolled tightly yet allow air to pass through freely. Used in rolling sushi, and also to cover freshly cooked foods or leftovers.

Sweet Brown Rice. A sweeter-tasting, more glutinous variety of rice. Used in mochi, ohagi, dumplings, and other dishes, it is often used in cooking for festive occasions.

Takuan. Daikon that is pickled in rice bran and sea salt. Sometimes called *takuwan*. Takuan is named after the Buddhist priest who invented this particular pickling method.

Taro. A type of potato with a thick, dark brown, hairy skin. Used as a vegetable or in the preparation of plasters for medicinal purposes. Also called *albi*.

Tekka. A condiment made from hatcho miso, sesame oil, burdock, lotus root, carrot, and ginger root, sautéed on a low flame for several hours.

Tempeh. A dish made from split soybeans, water, and a special bacteria that is allowed to ferment for several hours. Tempeh is eaten in Indonesia and Sri Lanka as a staple food. It is available prepacked, ready to prepare, in some natural-food stores. Rich in Vitamin B_{12} and protein.

Tofu. Soybean curd, made from soybeans and nigari (a coagulant taken from salt water). Used in soups, vegetable dishes, dressings, etc., tofu is high in protein. *See also* Dried Tofu.

Udon. Japanese noodles made from wheat, whole wheat, or whole-wheat and unbleached white flour. Udon generally have a lighter flavor than soba (buckwheat) noodles.

Umeboshi. Salty, pickled plums. Umeboshi plums stimulate the appetite and digestion and aid in maintaining an alkaline blood quality. Shiso leaves are usually added to the plums during pickling to impart a reddish color and natural flavoring.

Umeboshi Vinegar. A salty, sour vinegar made from umeboshi plums. Diluted with water and used in sweet-and-sour sauces, salads, salad dressings, etc.

Wakame. A long, thin, green sea vegetable used in making soups, salads, and vegetable dishes. High in protein, iron, and magnesium, wakame has a sweet taste and delicate texture and is especially good in miso soup.

Wasabi. A light green Japanese horseradish that is used in sushi or traditionally with raw fish (sashimi). Wasabi is a very hot spice.

Wheat Berries. The grains of whole wheat are often called wheat berries. Wheat berries are good when soaked and pressure-cooked together with brown rice.

Wheat Gluten. *See* Fu; Seitan.

Wild Rice. A wild grass that grows in water and is harvested by hand. Eaten traditionally by Native Americans in Minnesota and other areas.

Yinnie Syrup. A sweet, thick syrup made from rice and barley that is used in dessert cooking. This complex carbohydrate sweetener is preferable to simple sugars such as honey, maple syrup, and molasses, because the simple sugars are metabolized too quickly.

Yu-Dofu. A simmered tofu and vegetable dish served in a seasoned broth. This dish is popular throughout Japan and is ideal for autumn and winter evening meals. Served with a variety of dips, sauces, and garnishes.

INDEX

Aveline Kushi was born in 1923 in Yokata, Shimane-ken, Japan. She taught elementary school, junior high, and kindergarten upon graduating from teachers college in 1944. Aveline began her study of macrobiotics in 1950, under the guidance of George Ohsawa, and came to the United States the following year. She married Michio Kushi in 1952, and for the next ten years taught macrobiotic and natural-foods cooking in New York.

Michio and Aveline moved to Boston in 1965 and jointly established a variety of macrobiotic enterprises and educational ventures, including Erewhon, the leading distributor of natural and macrobiotic quality food; several macrobiotic restaurants, including Open Sesame; the *East West Journal* monthly; the East West Foundation; the Kushi Institute; and the Kushi Foundation. Aveline's classes in the Boston area attracted thousands of students over the years, and she gave seminars together with Michio in places such as England, France, Holland, Belgium, Germany, Italy, Spain, Portugal, Austria, Switzerland, Ireland, Costa Rica, Trinidad, Brazil, Hong Kong, and her native Japan.

The mother of five children—Lilian, Norio, Haruo, Yoshio, and Hisao—and the grandmother of four, Aveline authored several books including *The Quick and Natural Macrobiotic Cookbook* and *Aveline Kushi's Complete Guide to Macrobiotic Cooking*.

Wendy Esko was born in 1949, in upstate New York. She began macrobiotics in 1971 and moved to Boston two years later. She was married in 1974, and, together with her husband, Edward, and Michio and Aveline Kushi, helped develop the East West Foundation. She began giving cooking classes in 1976 and traveled to Japan for further study in 1978. Wendy currently works for Eden Foods, Inc., the largest natural and macrobiotic food distributor in North America. She lives in Clinton, Michigan. She co-authored several books including *Macrobiotic Cooking for Everyone* and *The Macrobiotic Cancer Prevention Cookbook*.

CLASSES AND FURTHER INFORMATION

Further information on implementing the macrobiotic diet can be obtained from the Kushi Institute, the leading macrobiotic educational center in the world. Founded in 1978 by Michio and Aveline Kushi, the Kushi Institute has offered guidance to individuals, families, and organizations for more than twenty years. To find out about classes and seminars, obtain more recipes, shop on line for macrobiotic foods, or to get the Kushi Institute newsletter, contact the Kushi Institute at the address below or visit them on line.

KUSHI INSTITUTE
PO Box 7
Becket, MA 01223
http://www.kushiinstitute.macrobiotics.org